To S

With respec[tion and ap?]
ciation for your work
towards our shared
goals.

Ronnie Shepard

Sept. 2010

RUNNING THE OBSTACLE COURSE TO SEXUAL AND REPRODUCTIVE HEALTH

RUNNING THE OBSTACLE COURSE TO SEXUAL AND REPRODUCTIVE HEALTH

Lessons from Latin America

BONNIE SHEPARD

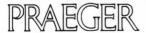

Westport, Connecticut
London

Library of Congress Cataloging-in-Publication Data

Shepard, Bonnie.
    Running the obstacle course to sexual and reproductive
  health : lessons from Latin America / Bonnie Shepard.
        p. cm.
    Includes bibliographical references and index.
    ISBN 0–275–97066–3 (alk. paper)
    1. Women's rights—Latin America. 2. Reproductive health—Latin America.
    3. Human rights advocacy—Latin America. I. Title.
    HQ1236.5.L37S54   2006
    306.7082'098–dc22   2006006638

British Library Cataloguing in Publication Data is available.

Library of Congress Catalog Card Number: 2006006638
ISBN: 0–275–97066–3

First published in 2006

Praeger Publishers, 88 Post Road West, Westport, CT 06881
An imprint of Greenwood Publishing Group, Inc.
www.praeger.com

Printed in the United States of America

The paper used in this book complies with the
Permanent Paper Standard issued by the National
Information Standards Organization (Z39.48–1984).

10 9 8 7 6 5 4 3 2 1

To José Barzelatto
(1926–2006)
An exceptional colleague, mentor and friend.
Your wisdom and commitment will continue to inspire us.

CONTENTS

PREFACE

I have spent most of my professional career since the 1980s working on reproductive and sexual health programs, but I first developed a passion for these issues while working on a project in Chile from 1972 to 1973 at the time of Salvador Allende's government. A multinational group of women friends got together to adapt *Our Bodies Ourselves*[1] for a Chilean audience, which was to appear in the government's women's magazine, *Paloma*.[2] I was in my early twenties at the time, and my interviews with low-income women in Mothers' Clubs on issues related to women's health and sexuality gave me a new understanding, grounded in Latin American realities, of how discrimination against women negatively affects their health, their experiences in the medical system, and their closest personal relationships. Although Chile's health system was in many ways superior to most public health systems in the Latin American region, I did not know that at the time. My observations of the lack of respect for birthing women and of sensitivity to their needs in assembly-line childbirth in the public hospitals shocked me profoundly.

During the 1980s at Pathfinder International in the Women's Programs Division, my colleagues and I worked hard to integrate women's rights perspectives into family planning and population programs.[3] Our division was very active in Latin America, a region of the world where feminist organizations were actively experimenting with new service models and advocating for women's rights. We also supported the integration of "women-in-development" programs with family planning services, to empower women economically while providing them choices in managing their fertility. Some of these USAID-funded efforts were greatly handicapped by having to "prove" that such integration made women more likely to use family planning.[4] In projects supported by private donors, Pathfinder supported seminal meetings of the Latin American feminist movement and the women's health movement. However, during the 1980s, most of these efforts remained marginal to the mainstream activities in the population and family planning field. At the global policy level and then at the national level, widespread acceptance of women's rights and gender equality as integral to all population and development efforts did not occur until the mid-1990s.

From 1992 to 1998, I was the program officer in charge of the Sexual and Reproductive Health Program in the Ford Foundation's Andean and Southern Cone Regional office. At that time, under the leadership of José Barzelatto and Margaret Hempel, the foundation's Reproductive Health Program played an important role in concert with many other organizations in stimulating the transformation of the population and family planning field. Both private foundations and governments supported the unprecedented involvement of civil society women's organizations in both extra-official and official deliberations in the mid-1990s at three key United Nations World Conferences: on human rights, population and development (ICPD), and women (FWCW).

The conference agreements—in particular that of ICPD—legitimized a shift in the goals of population programs from reduction of fertility to comprehensive health and well-being with regard to reproduction and sexuality, empowerment of women and involvement of men, and reproductive rights. With these new goals came new challenges—some related to active political and cultural resistance, and others to the translation of these broad goals into specific changes in program design, bureaucracies, and budgets. Reviewing this situation after the conferences, the Ford Foundation's Reproductive Health Latin American program officers[5] decided that we had two top priorities: to increase the effectiveness of advocacy to promote implementation of the ICPD Programme of Action, in particular at the national level, and to support any initiative that would provide guidance to both public and private programs on how to "operationalize" the goals of ICPD in health and population programs.

The idea for these four studies arose from my post–ICPD Ford Foundation experiences in the Andean and Southern Cone countries of Latin America, supporting programs that fit both priorities: women's rights and reproductive rights advocacy networks, as well as innovative pilot sexual and reproductive health programs. In the case of the advocacy programs, my experience as a donor was sobering, as both networks and individual NGOs confronted political resistance as well as internal tensions arising from the political costs of espousing often-controversial reproductive rights issues. In the case of innovative sexual and reproductive health programs that the foundation supported, political controversies at the national level and cultural resistance at the community level posed major obstacles to their implementation. However, the two programs analyzed in this book managed to overcome many of these obstacles. Therefore, my initial motivation for studying these programs arose from my enthusiasm for them and a belief that other similar programs could replicate or learn from these experiences, thus providing the needed guidance on implementing ICPD principles.

In 1998, I applied for and received an eighteen-month fellowship from the Ford Foundation, and a two-year fellowship from the David Rockefeller Center for Latin American Studies at Harvard University in order to carry out the research on which this book is based. I carried out two additional case studies of organizational changes within reproductive health services in Colombia and Ecuador that are not included in this collection.[6]

The view I had as a representative of a donor agency expanded greatly when I was no longer in that position and had the opportunity to conduct research on advocacy and programs. As I became more steeped in the participants' viewpoints on their experience, I began to collect data more systematically on how the political systems and conflicts surrounding the programs either hindered or facilitated their progress, and on how structures and incentives within institutions affected efforts to promote change.

The processes that promote political and/or organizational change are challenging to analyze. Resistance to change takes place from the global to the community level, with multiple actors in webs of influence, and tensions within and among institutions. The title "Running the Obstacle Course to Sexual and Reproductive Health" refers to the long-term complex nature of the process of change—with alternating progress and setbacks, and to how the concept of "citizenship" comes alive and encounters obstacles in advocacy and programs related to sexual and reproductive health. The process of change does not fit well into the logic of the donor-funded "projects" that I was accustomed to, and I began to see how the projects that I had supported were embedded in this long-term process. I became fascinated by disentangling the threads leading to change, analyzing the effects of different obstacles, and observing the ripple effects of interventions.

Reducing the complexity of lived experience to short, readable chapters in a book was the final challenge. These studies reflect only a fraction of the richness that I found in conversations with participants at all levels of the institutions involved. I had to abandon possible "stories" in the interests of coherence. Some of these appear in asides, boxes, and endnotes.

I collected most of the data over a two-year period from September 1998 to August 2000, mainly in Chile, Colombia, and Peru, with some updates through subsequent communications between 2001 and 2004 when I wrote the final versions. My experiences and opinions from twenty-five years of observation and conversations with advocates and program managers in sexual and reproductive health programs also inform the content of this book.

While particular historical experiences are never repeated, the nature of the resistance to sexual and reproductive health and rights is a global phenomenon, and I offer these studies to readers with the hope that the hypotheses and lessons arising from them will illuminate their experience.

the portraitist seeks to document and illuminate the complexity and detail of a unique experience or place, hoping that the audience will see themselves reflected in it. ... The portraitist is very interested in the single case because she believes that embedded in it the reader will discover resonant universal themes. The more specific, the more subtle the description, the more likely it is to evoke identification.[7]

NOTES

1. This book remains the main resource for the women's health movement in the United States, and has been translated and adapted into nineteen languages. For most of the Chilean project, the translation/adaptation group used the newsprint edition, before the very first Simon & Schuster edition appeared in 1973. The reference for the most recent edition is: Boston Women's Health Book Collective, *Our Bodies, Ourselves: A New Edition for a New Era*, New York: Touchstone/Fireside: Simon & Schuster, 2005. Currently, the author is co-chair of the Board of Directors of Our Bodies, Ourselves.

2. Only two copies of the manuscripts existed and both were lost. The authors' chapters were distributed among us in August 1973 after completion, and the chapters based on original research were lost as several authors fled the country or went into hiding at the time of the military coup in September 1973. The Editorial Quimantú copy was burned by the military along with most of the publications and manuscripts in the government publishing house's offices.

3. During the 1980s when I worked there, the organization's name was "Pathfinder Fund." Freya Olafson headed the division until 1986, when Pathfinder restructured and eliminated the thematic divisions. Judith Helzner was Program Associate until 1984.

4. See Helzner and Shepard 1997, for a discussion of this issue within the framework of promoting the feminist agenda within a population organization.

5. The other two program officers during the author's post–ICPD experiences were Lucille Atkin in Mexico and Sarah Costa in Brazil.

6. The case study in Colombia focused on the incorporation of sexuality counseling into the services of the IPPF/WH affiliate—Profamilia. " 'When I talk about sexuality, I use myself as an example': Sexuality counseling and family planning in Colombia" is published in *Responding to Cairo: Case studies of changing practice in reproductive health and family planning*, edited by Nicole Haberland and Diana Measham, New York: The Population Council. 2002. A second case study on incorporating gender issues and male involvement into the services of APROFE in Ecuador (also an IPPF/WH affiliate) was supported by a consultancy from IPPF/WH. *Addressing Gender*

Issues with Men and Couples: Involving Men in Sexual and Reproductive Health Services in APROFE, Ecuador, FXB Center Working Paper No. 13, Boston, MA: François-Xavier Bagnoud Center for Health and Human Rights, Harvard University. An article based on the paper is published in *International Journal of Men's Health,* Vol. 1, No. 1, 2005.

7. Sarah Lawrence Lightfoot, *The Art and Science of Portraiture,* San Francisco, CA: Jossey Bass.

ACKNOWLEDGMENTS

The research for this book, and the writing and translation of early drafts, was made possible by a fellowship from the Ford Foundation. I owe Alexander Wilde, the former representative at the foundation's Andean and Southern Cone office, a special thank you for encouraging me to develop the proposal to write this book. The David Rockefeller Center for Latin American Studies at Harvard University provided a welcoming working environment from September 1998 through September of 2000, during which time I conducted the bulk of the research and much of the writing for this book. Finally, my appointment as Visiting Scientist at the International Health and Human Rights Program of the François-Xavier Bagnoud Center for Health and Human Rights at Harvard School of Public Health has provided me with a collegial and supportive professional base since then, during the writing of the JOCAS and through two drafts of this book. Claudia Ordoñez and Mehera Dennison assisted in copy editing earlier drafts, and Catalina Forttes helped to edit this final version. Dr. José Barzelatto's helpful comments during the final peer review process gave me great encouragement, and helped to give the book its final shape.

I want to express my deepest gratitude to the people acknowledged below for their hospitality, their insights in personal interviews, their critiques on earlier drafts, and for responding to countless e-mails and telephone calls to update the studies and answer additional questions that arose during the writing.

Sofia Gruskin, editor of *Health and Human Rights*, provided invaluable edits and comments to Chapter 1 on the "double discourse." Special thanks also to Mala Htun, for her very useful comments on an earlier draft, and to Gaby Oré Aguilar, Maria Isabel Plata, Luisa Cabal, Elena Prada Salas, José Barzelatto, Josefina Hurtado, and Carmen Posada for their helpful comments on later drafts.

Kathleen Hamman and Jeffrey Stark, editors at the North-South Center Press, Dante B. Fascell Center, University of Miami, provided patient guidance and comments through many drafts of Chapter 2: the study of NGO advocacy networks. I thank colleagues who made insightful comments on earlier drafts of this chapter: Maruja Barrig, Carmen Barroso, Ana Güezmes, Amparo Claro, Susana Chiarotti, and an anonymous peer reviewer. Finally, I thank my friends and sisters in the NGO networks in Latin America, whose support and cooperation made the study possible. With great generosity, they submitted to extensive interviews and answered even the most intrusive questions. I offer them this study with a sense of humility because they are more familiar with the reality of their organizations than I can ever be. I hope that this analysis will be useful to them in their struggle to promote women's and reproductive rights.

The Population Council—in particular, Nicole Haberland, Diana Measham, and Deborah Rogow—provided support and extensive editing through numerous drafts of Chapter 3: the Consorcio Mujer study. Sylvia Madalengoitia of Centro de Estudios Sociales y Publicaciones (CESIP), the project coordinator, gave invaluable assistance through her overview of Consorcio Mujer from its inception, comments on an interim draft in Spanish, and by helping to coordinate my travel. Luz Maria Gallo and Virginia Agüero of Centro IDEAS in Piura, Magda Matteos and Rosario Salazar at Centro de Estudios y Promoción de la Mujer Amauta in Cusco, and Maribel Becerril of Centro de Estudios y Promoción Comunal del Oriente (CEPCO) in Tarapoto provided insights and introductions to the users and providers they had worked with, as did Ida Escudero of CESIP, Rocío Gutierrez of Movimiento Manuela Ramos, and Yngeborg Villena of Centro de la Mujer Peruana Flora Tristán in the Lima neighborhoods where they worked. I owe a special thank you to the health officials, service providers, and members of users' defense committees who gave generously of their time to talk about their experiences.

For Chapter 4—the study of the JOCAS in Chile—my heartfelt thanks and admiration go to those who generously shared their experiences and insights on the experiences of the JOCAS in interviews and cheerfully answered my e-mail queries: Paula Arriagada, Ximena Barria, Dr. Raquel Child, Germán González, Dr. Miguel Angel González, Magdalena Kleincsek, Irma Palma, Gabriela Pischedda, María de la Luz Silva, Rosario Solar, and Rodrigo Vera. I owe special thanks to Tim Frasca for his comments on the 2003 draft, and then again in 2004 for editing this chapter to get it down to a manageable size and scope. María de la Luz Silva provided extensive comments and historical information while correcting key errors in my draft. The richness of the information she provided deserves more attention than I could include here. Claudia Ordoñez, my former assistant at Harvard School of Public Health, helped with the transcription of tapes and notes. I wish to give a special mention to Alejandro Stuardo of Guernica Consultores for his commitment to young people and his insights. He shared his thoughts on the community-based program with me in early 2000 and died shortly thereafter in a tragic accident.

Deborah Carvalko, my editor at Praeger/Greenwood Publishing Group, deserves a special thank you for her patience as I struggled to find the time to finish this book in the midst of professional and family obligations.

My love and thanks to my husband David Holmstrom and our daughter Ana. They put up with my late nights and distraction as I fitted the research and writing of this book into the scarce spaces in my work and family life. Now I hope to have more time to cook cornbread and *caldo verde* and, as Ana always urges me, to "get a life."

ACRONYMS

CDD/LA: Catholics for the Right to Decide in Latin America (Católicas por el Derecho a Decidir, Latinoamérica). CDD groups are in Argentina Cordoba and Buenos Aires), Bolivia, Brazil, Chile, Colombia, and Mexico

CEDAW: Convention on the Elimination of All Forms of Discrimination Against Women

CEJIL: Center for Justice and International Law

CESIP: Center for Social Studies and Publications

CFFC: Catholics for a Free Choice (based in the United States) works with its sister organizations in the CDD/LA network on various global activities and exchanges

CLADEM: Comité de América Latina y el Caribe para la Defensa de los Derechos de la Mujer (Latin American and Caribbean Comittee for the Defense of Women's Rights)

CONASIDA: The Chilean government national AIDS program

CSO: Civil Society Organization

CWNSRR: Colombian Women's Network for Sexual and Reproductive Rights (Red Colombiana de Mujeres por los Derechos Sexuales y Reproductivos)

DEMUS: Office for the Defense of Women's Rights (Estudio para la Defensa de los Derechos de la Mujer)

EZLN: Zapatista Army for National Liberation (Ejército Zapatista de Liberación Nacional)

FGM: Female Genital Mutilation

FWCW: United Nations Fourth World Conference on Women

GBM: Green Belt Movement, Kenya

GIRE: Information Group for Reproductive Choice in Mexico (Grupo de Información sobre Reproducción Elegida)

ICASO: International Council of AIDS Service Organizations

ICMER: Chilean Institute for Reproductive Medicine (Instituto Chileno de Medicina Reproductiva)

ICPD: International Conference on Population and Development

IPPF/WHR: International Planned Parenthood Federation/Western Hemisphere Region

IUD: Intra Uterine Device

JOCAS: *Jornadas de Conversación sobre Afectividad y Sexualidad*, the "Conversation Workshops on Relationships and Sexuality" (Chile)

JOCCAS: The community-based model of JOCAS

LACWHN: Latin American and Caribbean Women's Health Network

MAM: Mass Women's Movement (Movimiento Amplio de Mujeres), Peru

MINEDUC: Chilean Ministry of Education

MINSA: Chilean Ministry of Health

MOH: Ministry of Health, Peru

NGO: Nongovernmental organization—usually used to refer to professionally staffed nonprofit organization, and not to community-based grassroots associations

OAS: Organization of American States

PRD: Democratic Revolutionary Party (Partido de la Revolución Democrática) Mexico

PROMUDEH: Ministry of Women's Promotion and Human Development (Ministerio de Promoción de la Mujer y del Desarrollo Humano)

PT: Workers' Party (Partido dos Trabalhadores) Brazil

RSMLAC: Red de Salud de Mujeres Latinoamericanas y del Caribe (name in Spanish of LACWHN)

RTI: Reproductive Tract Infection

SERNAM: Chilean National Women's Service

STI: Sexually Transmitted Infection
UNIFEM: United Nations Development Fund for Women
USAID: United States Agency for International Development
WEDO: Women's Environment and Development Organization
WHO: World Health Organization

INTRODUCTION

As Thomas Kuhn[1] noted, paradigm shifts in science are fiercely contested, and stem from a build-up of discoveries and new knowledge that changes the fundamental theoretical underpinnings of a scientific discipline. Paradigm shifts in public policy are equally contested, but are usually related to a shift in political power structures and/or policy goals as a result of mounting pressure from diverse coalitions and actors. At the beginning of a paradigm shift in public policy, when the first definite steps in a new direction tip the balance away from traditional paths or structures, those who advocated for the shift are jubilant. A momentous victory has been won, and it seems certain that the next steps will follow inevitably in the new direction. The enemy—outdated and hidebound tradition—has been defeated, and momentum is on the side of innovation. In those initial heady moments, few foresee the obstacle course that lies ahead to maintaining the new direction, translating it into concrete changes, and overcoming resistance to change at all levels in society. The International Conference on Population and Development (ICPD) in 1994 was such a moment for global population policy, as the overall goals shifted from fertility reduction and population control to comprehensive reproductive health and well-being, women's empowerment, and reproductive rights.

When such paradigm shifts start at the global policy level, the new general goals subsume diverse issues. For example, the goal of women's empowerment entails attention to issues such as discrimination against women in education and employment, gender-based violence, female genital mutilation (FGM), and early marriage. Following the shift in overall goals, the next challenge is to promote attention to these more specific issues, so that UN and donor agencies, civil society organizations, and leaders in governments will translate these important policy gains into changes in international and national laws, policies, and programs.

This challenge is not a simple matter, because important advances often lead to backlash and resistance of equal or greater proportions. In the case of sexual and reproductive health, there are well-financed organizations supporting the backlash globally. While the most publicized face of the backlash occurs in UN meetings such as the "ICPD+10" meetings in 2004, less evident but equally intense resistance occurs within agencies, governments, and at the community level. Finding ways to overcome or circumvent this resistance is a major task for advocacy groups and for sexual and reproductive health programs.

Meeting this resistance requires a process of political and cultural change in organizations and communities; until that happens, the new laws or policies remain rhetoric that have not yet become reality. For example, both the UN system and many governments now have clear policies against gender and racial discrimination, and yet behaviors, attitudes, or traditions that discriminate against women and/or ethnic minorities are present in most countries. Additional examples are all too easy to identify. Advocates in many countries have worked with national decision makers to secure the passage of new laws against gender-based violence, FGM, or early marriage. However, flouting of these laws will continue to be widespread until communities undergo cultural change that increases support for these new norms. Worldwide, there are many successful examples of bringing about the necessary cultural changes in institutions and communities. However, traditional cultural frameworks and beliefs are deep-rooted and often operate subconsciously. Therefore, attempts to change them have to be participatory and require a long-term view. Combating discrimination in institutions and communities entails bringing the discriminatory norms and practices to the surface, subjecting them to conscious scrutiny in the light of day, and then promoting cultural change.

There are multiple cultural, intellectual, and political processes at different levels in a given society or in the global policy arena that stimulate a paradigm shift. No matter which sector in society takes the lead in a paradigm shift—whether political elites or "mass culture"—the work of translating new principles into concrete policy or behavioral changes at different levels of society is littered with obstacles and setbacks as the lead sector attempts all means at its disposal to turn the tide. Sometimes influential organizations—corporations, foundations, universities, NGOs, or government agencies—promote a new policy goal supported by a progressive (or conservative) minority; they might or might not have sufficient influence on others to bring the rest of society on board. Sometimes global or national policies lag behind civil society attitudes and behaviors, especially when the policy relates to widespread practices that contravene the teachings of influential religions. The so-called sexual revolution in Europe and the United States in the 1960s is a good example of this type of shift, as is the case of divorce in Chile, discussed in Chapter 1.

The four studies presented in this book examine this obstacle course to social change, post-ICPD, in Latin America. Two of the studies focus on advocacy initiatives and/or organizations. They aim to illuminate the facilitating factors as well as the obstacles to advocacy for policy change to fulfill the human right to sexual and reproductive health, both in the national context and within advocacy organizations. The next two studies highlight the successful yet short-lived experiences of two programs in Peru and Chile in the late 1990s in the health and education sectors respectively. The programs translated human rights principles of reproductive rights, gender equity, and citizen participation into concrete program models, while encountering obstacles that ultimately brought about their demise. All four studies suggest ways forward for advocacy groups, schools, and health services.

To set the stage for reading these studies, this introduction will describe in more detail the shifts in the mid-1990s in the population field. Following will be a brief description of each study. Chapter 5, the conclusion to this book, will discuss the crosscutting issues in the studies: contested sexual and reproductive health issues, democratization and citizen participation, organizational change processes, and project versus program approaches.

THE TRANSFORMATION OF THE POPULATION FIELD: INCORPORATING HUMAN RIGHTS AND GENDER ISSUES

Leading Up to ICPD

Many advances in policy, international law, global social movements, and research related to population, health, human rights, and gender issues led up to ICPD during the two decades that span from the first UN Conference on Population and Development in 1974 to the watershed moment of ICPD in 1994. Four important trends leading up to ICPD will be discussed here. First, the definitions of reproductive health and of reproductive rights that formed the guiding axis of the ICPD Programme of Action were based on two principles of health embodied in the first paragraphs of the World Health Organization's (WHO) constitution. The first WHO principle defines "health" as "a state of complete physical, mental, and social well-being and not merely the absence of disease or infirmity," thus leading to broader, more comprehensive approaches to health that include, but are not limited to, the field of medicine. The second principle embodies "the enjoyment of the highest attainable standard of health" as "a fundamental right of every human being without distinction of race, religion, political belief, economic or social condition."[2] Almost thirty years later, the International Covenant on Economic, Social, and Cultural Rights (1976) further affirmed a comprehensive rights-based framework for health that addresses the social and economic determinants of ill health and inequities in the enjoyment of health.

Second, during the same two decades, the worldwide expansion of activism in favor of women's rights constituted another potent influence on the population field. During the International Women's Decade from 1975 to 1985, women's activists from all continents met at "NGO Forums" at three UN conferences. The growing international women's health movement was particularly active at these conferences. When these women's organizations examined the premises underpinning population control programs, they observed that the overriding goal of fertility control led to coercive practices, disregard for women's health, and lack of concern for women's right to full informed choice in reproductive matters. Prominent examples were the coercive sterilization programs (targeted at both men and women) in India, and family planning experiments that introduced new contraceptives without sufficient evidence on health risks, such as the widespread marketing in the early 1970s of the unsafe IUD—the Dalkon Shield—which caused alarming numbers of cases of infection, infertility, and death worldwide.

Third, opposition to the prevailing paradigm of population control came from the socialist and communist political tradition, whose adherents objected strongly to the standard argument that unchecked population control was causing widespread poverty in developing countries. They pointed to inequities in the world economy and national economies as the main driving force behind poverty, and levied charges of genocide and imperialism against Northern politicians seeking to reduce the numbers of their dark-skinned neighbors to the South. This trend in the opposition dominated the debates at the First World Conference on Population and Development in Bucharest in 1974.

Fourth, in the environmental movement—traditionally allied with population control agencies—dissenting voices began to point to consumption patterns in industrialized low-fertility countries rather than rising numbers in high-fertility countries as the main culprit in global environmental degradation.

In summary, progressive trends in the UN system, in international human rights law, in the women's rights and environmental movements, and among socialist countries and leading intellectuals converged in the 1970s and through the 1990s to undermine the paradigm of population control.

However, research within population organizations and agencies also contributed to the shifts ushered in by ICPD. Researchers in the population field noted that in many countries, simply supplying family planning services did not lead to use of contraception, and began to examine the barriers to "demand" for family planning. The more demographers and other social scientists examined the dynamics behind women's patterns of high fertility, the more they found poverty, gender issues, cultural valuation of high fertility, fear and distrust of the medical establishment, and lack of social security systems as the driving forces. The association between increased educational levels for women and lower fertility was established by numerous studies. The Population Council was in the vanguard of efforts to introduce the "users' perspective" in concepts of quality in family planning programs, in order to afford women respectful treatment and full informed choice, and in the process, improve demand.[3] Several other major population agencies—including USAID—experimented with programs designed to raise women's status while providing access to family planning education and services, to see whether raising status affected demand.[4] In other words, from within the population field, the realization of the need for a more rights-based and comprehensive approach was growing.

In the 1990s, two United Nations conferences preceded and followed ICPD, and both significantly increased the legitimacy of efforts to advance women's rights based on the Convention on the Elimination of All Forms of Discrimination against Women, which entered into force in 1981. The consensus agreements in the World Conference on Human Rights in Vienna in 1993 and the Fourth World Conference on Women (FWCW) in Beijing in 1995[5] made important advances in global policy, including greater recognition of women's rights as human rights and of "domestic" violence against women as a violation of women's rights. ICPD transformed the population field through its focus on women's rights, incorporating "women's empowerment" into the central agenda of population and development programs.[6] All three conferences included an unprecedented level of civil society organizations' (CSOs) involvement, both in official meetings and in parallel NGO Fora.[7] This involvement and the policy changes promoted by CSOs were inextricably linked to the broader social changes advanced by democratization movements from the late 1960s through the 1990s: respect for human rights, acceptance of diversity, elimination of discrimination, and promotion of citizenship and empowerment.

The 1994 ICPD Programme of Action put human beings' welfare and rights at the center of all development and population policies. ICPD focused on three basic guiding principles: comprehensive sexual and reproductive health, women's empowerment, and respect for individuals' and couples' reproductive rights. In 1995, the Beijing Platform for Action included a fuller range of issues central to women's empowerment and rights, and in its language even advanced slightly in the area of rights to sexual health, defined by ICPD (7.3) as "the enhancement of life and personal relations, and not merely...care related to reproduction and STDs." The Platform for Action further elaborated:

96. The human rights of women include their right to have control over and decide freely and responsibly on matters related to their sexuality, including sexual and reproductive health, free of coercion, discrimination and violence. Equal relationships between women and men in matters of sexual relations and reproduction, including full respect for the integrity of the person, require mutual respect, consent and shared responsibility for sexual behavior and its consequences.[8]

The term "sexual rights" has never made its way into any conference consensus agreement or international human rights treaty, but the ICPD Programme of Action states that the concept of "reproductive health" includes sexual health. By that same logic, "reproductive rights" includes the right to information, education, and services related to both reproductive and sexual health.

Obstacles to Implementing ICPD Principles: Resistance and Confusion

As mentioned above, a strong backlash and resistance to one or more of the main ICPD principles is perhaps the most important obstacle to converting the principles into concrete changes in national programs and policies. Commitment to gender equity and to fulfillment of human rights is necessary to protect health, but these principles often run counter to the dominant norms in a given culture. The first two chapters illustrate how advocacy for legal divorce and safe, legal abortion to reduce maternal deaths run into political resistance arising from dominant religious and cultural norms. In Chapter 3, Consorcio Mujer's focus on users' rights and participation went against the grain of traditionally hierarchical Peruvian health services. In Chapter 4 on the JOCAS in Chile, the uncensored free expression of the students in a participatory sex education program erupted into the public domain through the media, igniting public controversies and political pressures from religious leaders to shut down the program.

Another important source of resistance was and is bureaucratic. Reorganization in bureaucracies is often chaotic and conflictive. Managers of vertical programs in government or international donor agencies—maternal-child health, family planning, STIs, and in the 1990s HIV/AIDS—have jobs and budgets to defend. Attempts to unite two or more programs under one umbrella to create a comprehensive sexual and reproductive health program can unseat senior officials, create lay-offs, and cause logistical headaches. Not surprisingly, even within population agencies that officially endorsed ICPD, many senior managers were resistant to the loss of an exclusive focus on family planning.

Another obstacle arises from uncertainty about how to implement ICPD principles. Any new and pioneering direction has no road map to follow. Those who support the new paradigm in theory still need to figure out how to integrate these principles into their policies and programs. How does one transform the fundamental philosophy and goals behind a program? Is it a different configuration of services and activities? If so, which ones? How do work plans and procedures change? If the needed change is attitudinal among staff, how do we bring that about? How does one deal with resistance from one's own staff, from other stakeholders? Do we need new incentives and performance indicators? What are the budgetary implications? How can we be more comprehensive within the same budget? Reproductive health includes so many issues; how can we prioritize? How does one measure success?

Attempting to answer these questions, program after program reinvented the wheel when experimenting with integration of the principles accepted at ICPD. In many countries, family planning programs changed their label to "reproductive health," but did little different except for adding single services such as cervical cancer screening. Decision-makers in many agencies either actively resisted or threw up their hands in bewilderment when asked to incorporate a "gender perspective" or a "rights-based" approach.

In Latin America, the pilot programs pioneered by feminist organizations in the 1980s and early 1990s constituted a promising source of guidance, because they pre-figured the principles agreed on at ICPD and FWCW of comprehensive sexual and reproductive health, women's empowerment, and respect for women's and reproductive rights. However, these feminist efforts tended to be short-lived projects, or small-scale programs that were hard to "scale up," that is, to bring to a national or regional level with mass coverage at a reasonable cost.

Reproductive and sexual health advocates and program managers have been engaged in this dual challenge of advocacy to counter resistance and guidance to assist implementation ever since ICPD. There have been many successes. Most recently, the countries of the world resoundingly reaffirmed the Programme of Action in the ICPD+10 meetings in 2004, despite intense lobbying by the U.S. delegation and a handful of other countries. However, within agencies and organizations, whether due to failure to buy into the new principles or confusion about how to proceed, or both, delays and resistance are rife in the organizational change process. Often, the two obstacles are related. The answers to the questions that arise are complex enough that confusion is an easy excuse for failure to act. Initial steps to implement rights-based approaches can incite resistance among the staff, leading managers to decide to abandon the effort. Many decision-makers use the new consensus rhetoric, but are not completely convinced of these new principles. In this situation, it is convenient to focus on the difficulties, complaining that the process of implementing these principles is too complex and costly, or too difficult to grasp.

However, the confusion is real, not just a pretext; it must be addressed. We are all "bush-whacking" in uncharted territory and the way ahead is not always clear. Both the convinced and the unconvinced express the need for "tools," "guidelines," "indicators," and "road maps" to help them implement the principles embodied in these new phrases: "gender perspective," "rights-based programming," "sexual and reproductive health," or "male involvement."

Efforts to address these two obstacles to implementing ICPD—resistance and the need for guidance—form the two axes for this book. Putting ICPD principles into practice in programs usually requires both advocacy with decision-makers and experimentation with new models and strategies at the program level. Ongoing staff training and new incentives are necessary in order to effect the sustained transformation.

DESCRIPTION OF THE STUDIES—FOCUS AND METHODOLOGY

These studies analyze experiences in countries in the Southern Cone and Andean Region of Latin America, where the author lived and worked from 1992–1998. Corresponding to the main types of challenges post-ICPD, the four chapters fall into two categories: (1) studies of the political and organizational dynamics of sexual and reproductive health advocacy, and (2) studies of innovative experiments in implementing ICPD principles along with the rights-based mandate to enhance the participation of young people and women in the programs that affect their lives.

The Advocacy Studies

Chapter 1: The "Double Discourse" on Sexual and Reproductive Rights. This study analyzes the cultural and religious norms that pose formidable obstacles to sexual and reproductive health advocacy in Latin America. The article argues that societies accommodate conflicting views on sexuality and reproduction with a "double discourse system" that causes a disjunction between the public and private spheres. Official speech and policies on sexual and reproductive health must be based in religious dogma, leading to failure to protect the health of a country's inhabitants. On the other hand, governments tolerate unofficial and often illegal mechanisms that expand private sexual and reproductive choices, so long as they stay out of the public eye. These unofficial mechanisms for expanded choice are mostly available to the middle and upper classes, leading to inequities in enjoyment of the basic right to health. The examples of divorce policy in Chile and abortion policy in Colombia and Chile are highlighted to illustrate how this "chasm" between public discourse and private actions operates in practice, and who is harmed by it. The article concludes by discussing the implications of this system for rights advocacy, and provides some suggestions for reducing the political costs of transgression in countries characterized by this system.

The study is mainly based on findings from a literature review that included published sources as well as a corpus of unpublished sources: conference papers, agency-funded evaluation reports, and unpublished theses. The study also draws on the author's reflections on her experiences in the 1980s and 1990s with advocacy initiatives in Latin America. Conversations with colleagues in Chile and Colombia and several readers of first drafts added valuable content to the article.

Chapter 2: NGO Advocacy Networks in Latin America. This study analyzes the experiences during the 1990s of thirteen Latin American regional and national networks of nongovernmental organizations that advocate for sexual and reproductive rights and women's rights.

The questions guiding this study arose from the author's reflections on her experiences with these networks while working at the Ford Foundation. The networks had trouble constituting themselves as actors with a public voice in the national arena, and the study aimed to analyze the reasons for their difficulties. The questions relate to the relationship between the political advocacy role of these networks and their governance structure, facilitating factors or obstacles to their advocacy, and the most appropriate advocacy strategies for such networks.

The study highlights several dilemmas. Feminist networks reacting against authoritarian structures often strive for consensus decision-making and nonhierarchical structures, limiting their ability to take decisive action on controversial sexual and reproductive health advocacy issues. Analysis of problems related to membership, decision-making, and leadership structures provides some helpful insights for other advocacy networks. The effect of financial pressures on struggling NGOs limited their ability to take controversial stances, as did expansion of membership to enhance diversity. The chapter discusses and analyzes the successes of these NGO networks and the problems they faced, leading to suggestions for other advocacy networks in the often-contentious spheres of sexual and reproductive health and rights.

The study draws on an extensive literature search on networks, the women's movement, and political coalitions, as well as the author's personal experiences as a donor to the networks. These sources are complemented by in-depth semistructured interviews with five regional and eight national networks; some of these are group interviews, and others individual interviews with the network coordinators. National networks from Chile, Peru, Colombia, and Mexico were interviewed. Networks of grassroots, provincial (outside of the capital) or rural organizations are not represented in the study.

The Program Case Studies

These programs in Peru and Chile experimented with rights-based approaches based on goals of women's and young people's empowerment. The interventions challenged the traditional hierarchical systems of Peruvian health clinics and Chilean schools, while promoting women's and young people's access to vital health information and services. In different ways, both programs aimed to change the culture of the institutions where the intervention took place.

Chapter 3: "Let's Be Citizens, Not Patients!" This study of the Consorcio Mujer program in Peru analyzes the experiences of a consortium of women's movement organizations in an innovative four-city experiment that promoted respect for users' rights through involving women's community organizations in evaluation of quality of public health services. The consortium explicitly promoted a model of women's citizenship that countered the traditional paternalistic, and often abusive, model of provider-client relationships in the health services in Peru. The consortium conducted needs assessments of quality of care, involving both health providers and community women. These assessments fed into training workshops on quality of care and users' rights for both health providers and community members, and the development of proposals for quality improvements for each health center. The project aimed to achieve a more equal sustained relationship between the two groups through the establishment of Users' Committees among community organizations, and Quality of Care Committees in the health centers.

The study illustrates the tensions and dynamics that arise between community members and health service providers when women strive to become "citizens, and not patients," exercising community oversight of health services. The findings suggest some factors that would facilitate similar efforts in other locations, and help create sustainable channels for dialogue between health services and the communities they serve.

In the Peruvian study, the author conducted semistructured interviews with the NGO coordinators, leaders of the participating women's organizations, and health professionals at the six project sites during a two-week period in December 1998. These interviews are complemented by subsequent conversations with the Consorcio Mujer leaders during subsequent trips to Peru in 1999 and 2000, notes from an observation of an all-day meeting in Piura in 1997, and visits to all the other five sites between 1994 and 1997 while the author still worked at the Ford Foundation. These sources of data are complemented by literature on the health system in Peru at the time of the study, and studies published by Peruvian women's NGOs.

Chapter 4: "Conversations and Controversies: A Sexuality Education Program in Chile." This study describes a government-sponsored sex education program in Chilean schools and communities: the "Conversation Workshops on Relationships and Sexuality," or JOCAS (the acronym in Spanish). The case shows how a participatory program with empowerment goals for adolescents adapted to a socially conservative context when faced with intense public controversy, and scaled up to include half (600) of all of the secondary schools in Chile. The program consists of the promotion of informal and uncensored conversations among students, and then among students and parents, complemented by contact with community resource people who answer students' questions on sexual and reproductive health issues. The study highlights the strengths as well as the limitations of this highly decentralized and participatory model. It analyzes factors limiting parent participation and suggests possible mechanisms to ensure students' access to comprehensive sexual and reproductive health information in locally controlled schools. Finally, the study examines the political dynamics and tensions that contributed to the demise of the program.

The JOCAS experience illustrates how controversies surrounding adolescent sexual and reproductive health programs wear down political will. This experience is repeated in diverse forms in almost every country, finally resulting in a nearly worldwide failure of governments to fulfill their obligation to protect the health of vulnerable young people.

For the study of the JOCAS, the author conducted face-to-face and telephonic semistructured interviews with professionals and government officials closely involved with the design and implementation of the JOCAS from mid-1998 through 2003. In 1998, the author observed one JOCAS training session involving teachers, parents, and students from several schools. Numerous e-mail exchanges with these professionals supplemented the interviews, as did review of evaluation reports, manuals, and newspaper articles.[9] Although none of those interviewed by the author were at the school level (students, teachers, administrators, or parents), the study draws on earlier evaluations that interviewed and surveyed school-level stakeholders. Through her program at the Ford Foundation, the author supported the evaluation study of the first thirty pilot schools in 1995 and 1996, and attended meetings related to the JOCAS in the period from 1995–1997.

RUNNING THE OBSTACLE COURSE

Globally and within most countries, there is progress in fulfillment of the human right to sexual and reproductive health. In 2005, from the author's vantage point in the United States, these rights seem particularly threatened, but the countries of the world resoundingly defeated the U.S. administration's efforts to roll back the ICPD agreements in the ICPD+10 meetings in 2004.

Revealing the point of view of participants, these studies shed light on attempts to address both the resistance fulfilling the basic human right to sexual and reproductive health and the need for guidance in how to do so. The lessons from the experience of these advocates and programs in Latin America should help others to turn the rhetoric of ICPD into the reality of policies and programs. Progress on fulfilling sexual and reproductive rights will always suffer setbacks and obstacles, many of which are placed on the course by well-organized and well-financed conservative groups. Nonetheless, in this obstacle course, the overall direction of the runners is forward. May this book contribute to their progress.

NOTES

1. Thomas Kuhn, *The Structure of Scientific Revolutions*, Chicago: University of Chicago Press, 1962.

2. Original text of the WHO constitution accessed on October 21, 2005: http://w3.whosea.org/LinkFiles/About_SEARO_const.pdf. An interesting discussion of amendments since 1948 can be found in: Dr. U Than Sein, "Constitution of the World Health Organization and Its Evolution," *Regional Health Forum*, Volume 6, No. 1, 2002; accessed on October 21, 2005: http://w3.whosea.org/rhf/rhf6–1/7whoconstitution.htm.

3. See Judith Bruce 1990. Her framework was disseminated widely, leading to a body of literature on the subject.

4. See Helzner and Shepard 1990 and 1997. The experiments suffered from various design flaws, including too short a time frame and too few participants, and so they did not contribute to the literature on the link between women's status and fertility patterns.

5. The Vienna Declaration and Programme of Action A/CONF.157/23, July 12, 1993; accessed in June 2005: http://www.unhchr.ch/huridocda/huridoca.nsf/(Symbol)/A.CONF.157.23.En?OpenDocument; The Programme of Action of the International Conference on Population and Development, Report of the International Conference on Population and Development, September 5–13, 1994, UN Doc. A/CONF.171/13; accessed in June 2005: http://www.unfpa.org/icpd/docs/index.htm; The Platform for Action from the Beijing Conference A/CONF.177/20/REV.1; accessed in June 2005: http://www.un.org/womenwatch/confer/beijing/reports/.

6. See the chapter on the international women's movement in Keck and Sikkink 1998, for a comprehensive description of this historical process.

7. The literature on the role of women's and other civil society NGOs in the ICPD and FWCW conferences and in the follow-up conference five years later is vast. The websites of The Women's Environment and Development Organization (WEDO), the Center for Reproductive Rights, the International Women's Health Coalition, ISIS Internacional, the Latin American and Caribbean Women's Health Network, CLADEM, the United Nations Population Fund, and the UN "Women Watch" site all contain useful articles, summaries, and access to other publications.

8. The Platform for Action from the Beijing Conference op. cit.

9. One respondent provided copies of the relevant Chilean newspaper articles from 1996–1997. Sources for other articles are mainly from the Internet.

1

THE "DOUBLE DISCOURSE" ON SEXUAL AND REPRODUCTIVE RIGHTS IN LATIN AMERICA: THE CHASM BETWEEN PUBLIC POLICY AND PRIVATE ACTIONS

The international policy arena today is marked by strong clashes of values with regard to sexuality and reproduction. This chapter[1] will examine how political controversies affect citizens' ability to exercise sexual and reproductive rights in Latin America, with examples from several countries, but focusing mainly on Chile. This study describes how societies accommodate conflicting views on sexuality and reproduction via a "double discourse system," which maintains the status quo in repressive or negligent public policies while expanding private sexual and reproductive choices behind the scenes. Two specific examples—divorce law in Chile and abortion advocacy in Colombia and Chile—will highlight how this breach between public discourse and private actions operates in practice, and who is harmed by it. The chapter will conclude by discussing the implications of this system for rights advocacy.

In Latin America and throughout the world, general consensus exists among governments on the now-standard phrases that summarize reproductive rights in the Programme of Action of the International Conference on Population and Development (ICPD), held in Cairo in 1994:

[Reproductive rights refers to] the basic right of all couples and individuals to decide freely and responsibly the number, spacing and timing of their children, and to have the information and means to do so, and the right to attain the highest standard of reproductive and sexual health. [Reproductive rights] also includes [couples and individuals'] right to make decisions concerning reproduction free of discrimination, coercion and violence, as expressed in human rights documents.[2]

In Latin America, as in many other regions, certain concrete implications of these principles of consensus are vehemently disputed at all levels, from the family to the central government. Do these rights extend to adolescents—that is, do adolescents count as "couples and individuals"? In the two rounds of post-ICPD meetings in 1999 and 2004, whenever issues related to adolescents' access to reproductive health services arose, conservative country delegations opposed these provisions, arguing that parents' rights supersede those of adolescents.

Other implications of reproductive rights arouse controversy. If women have the right to decide freely on the number and spacing of their children, doesn't that entail the right to safe abortion services? This is certainly the most publicized conflict in the reproductive rights field, so much so that all too often the term "reproductive rights" is reduced to the issue of abortion in the public mind. It should also be noted that while there finally appears to be some consensus that sexual violence and coercion are violations of basic human rights, many conservative groups remain opposed to the term "sexual rights," which they believe will lead to recognition of freedom of sexual orientation as a right.

REPRESSIVE PUBLIC LAWS AND EXPANDED PRIVATE OPTIONS: SEXUAL AND REPRODUCTIVE RIGHTS IN LATIN AMERICA

The political climate surrounding sexual and reproductive rights is characterized by a worldwide increase in religious fundamentalism on the one hand and cultural globalization on the other, which has exacerbated preexisting political and cultural divisions. In Latin America, the majority of citizens identify as Roman Catholic, and the church is the main force against full recognition of sexual and reproductive rights. As in European countries with a dominantly Catholic tradition and among Catholics in the United States, most studies show that in practice Latin American Catholics do not follow the official teachings of the church on the use of contraception and abortion.[3] The increasing strength of hard-line factions over the past twenty years has resulted in growing rigidity in the church's position on these issues and increasing repression of dissident views within Catholic institutions.[4] Although the channels through which the Roman Catholic hierarchy exercises its political influence are often hidden from public view, the visible result is policies that deny reproductive and sexual rights to citizens—policies that seem to become ever more deeply entrenched in a polarized political climate.

How do Latin American countries accommodate the sharp divisions in public opinion on these issues and the universal and often pressing need for individuals and couples to exercise freedom of decision-making in sexuality and reproduction? In many cultures, escape valves allow private accommodations that sidestep repressive policies, leaving the official legal and/or religious norms untouched while reducing the social and political pressure for policy advances.

This type of societal rift between public stands and private actions also operates at the level of the individual. Rosalind Petchesky has discussed women's private strategies to expand their reproductive choices:

As our fieldwork progressed ... we found that the two extremes of outright resistance and passive accommodation are much rarer than the kinds of complicated, subtle reproductive and sexual strategies that most of our respondents adopt in order to achieve some degree of autonomy and at the same time maintain their place in the family and community. ... [A woman] may see no contradiction whatsoever in both acting against a particular norm and speaking in deference to it. Indeed, accommodation in practice often means a non-confrontational or conciliatory way of achieving one's wishes or sense of right.[5]

The Double Discourse System

A recurrent theme within the Latin American countries with which the author is most familiar—Colombia, Peru, Chile, and Argentina[6]—is the "double discourse" (*doble discurso*). This phrase, usually applied to individuals, is widely understood to signify the art of espousing traditional and repressive sociocultural norms publicly, while ignoring—or even participating in—the widespread flouting of these norms in private. This chapter expands the use of the term "double discourse" to signify a political and cultural system, not just an agglomeration of individuals privately "sinning." Thanks to the ubiquity of the double discourse, in most Latin American countries the reproductive and sexual choices open to citizens are much wider than what the official policies would lead one to believe. At the heart of this system lies the chasm between public discourse, upholding traditional religious precepts that limit individual choices, and unofficial private discourses—in conversations, interior monologues, and the confessional—that rationalize or ask forgiveness for transgressions. These private individual discourses are complemented by social and political mechanisms—in various forms such as laws or interpretations of laws, common practices, or clandestine services—that provide an escape valve from repressive norms and make expanded choices possible. The primary features of the double discourse system, then, are the following:

- For historical and political reasons, the *hierarchies of a hegemonic religion exercise considerable influence over state policies,* imposing the religion's moral codes on legal norms. The distinction between immorality and criminality is blurred.

- *The official discourse and policies uphold highly restrictive norms based in religious doctrine*, and assume a sacred and inviolable character. These norms violate citizens' sexual and reproductive rights through repression or coercion and/or by preventing the state from fulfilling its obligation to protect the health of its citizens.

- *There are always political costs attached to espousing a change in the norm, which is sacred.* Public officials and civil society organizations come under attack when they publicly defend the legitimacy of the sexual or reproductive right in question or when they attempt to reform the policies.

- Individual practices that flout the norm are widespread, as are informal or illegal social and political mechanisms that make them possible. These mechanisms constitute an escape valve that expands citizens' sexual and reproductive choices. However, because the mechanisms are illegal or unofficial, neither availability, safety (in the case of services), nor protections of basic rights are guaranteed. Examples of such mechanisms include legal loopholes for marriage annulments when divorce is not legal, and clandestine abortion clinics.

- The worst consequences of the restrictive policies fall on low-income sectors and on groups that are disadvantaged, discriminated against, or marginalized in other ways, for example, ethnic minorities, single mothers, inhabitants of rural areas, and homosexual men and women. Political elites—generally from high-income sectors—usually do not suffer the worst consequences of the restrictive laws.

- *The high political costs attached to efforts for reform*, the political disenfranchisement of the groups that feel the worst consequences of the restrictive policies, and the existence of informal mechanisms that expand choice—all lead to a lack of political will for reform. Public debate exposing the system can lead to increased repression and limits on the informal mechanisms, thus restricting choice in practice and creating ethical dilemmas for advocates of reform.

Clearly, this chasm between public norms restricting individual rights and private discourses and mechanisms expanding them is not limited to the area of sexual and reproductive rights. So many sociocultural taboos and restrictions lie in this realm, however, that in Latin American popular usage *el doble discurso* generally refers to sexual and reproductive matters. In fact, the term "double discourse" is somewhat misleading, because its essence is that private actions deviating from the norm, even if they are almost universally practiced, are not favored with any *public* discourse at all that defends their legitimacy. The *private* discourse does not usually defend the sexual and reproductive rights that contravene these traditional norms; rather, it rationalizes individual actions or explains them in terms of weakness and sin.

Doble discurso is a fitting nonjudgmental label arising from these predominantly Catholic cultures, since the closest words in English for this phenomenon—for example, "hypocritical," "deceptive," "two-faced," and "duplicitous"—are harsh in their judgments. The polarized debates that often coexist with double discourse systems beget severe judgments. In the debates about sex education in Chile, the reformers believe that they are simply recognizing the reality and risks of adolescent sexual behavior, while their opponents are "hypocrites" who hide their heads in the sand. Likewise, those opposing the public health approach to sex education accuse the reformers of being "permissive" and promoting "promiscuity."[7] It might be fair to say that a double discourse system is built into Catholic cultures in those countries where for a variety of historical and political reasons the church has great influence on the state. In these countries, most of which are in Latin America, public officials often feel compelled to uphold the church's teachings publicly although they know that actions at variance with the teachings are common.[8] Catholics view this attitude not as hypocritical, but rather as upholding an ideal to which many, including oneself, fail to measure up, for reasons that God will understand and forgive.

Similar to the women described above by Petchesky, both Catholic women and the clergy make their personal peace with private choices that flout official norms. Clergy at the grassroots level are often more empathetic and flexible than the hierarchy. As the hierarchy often "silences" clergy who speak out publicly against the church's repressive norms on sexuality and reproduction, their support for individuals' forbidden reproductive and sexual behaviors usually takes place in the private realm of conversations and the confessional.[9] A little-known study in Colombia on the attitudes of Catholic women and Catholic priests on abortion[10] showed that most priests give absolution in the confessional to women who have had abortions, despite recent edicts urging priests to excommunicate women who have had abortions. For their part, Catholic women interviewed in abortion clinics made a de facto distinction between the public notion of mortal sin and the private spiritual notion of an understanding deity. Although they recognized that abortion is a sin, they stated that their relationship with God was not in any way ruptured by their actions, which arose from extreme hardship and necessity.

The examples of divorce law in Chile and abortion advocacy in Colombia and Chile will demonstrate these features of the double discourse system. Both illustrate how policymakers are willing to turn a blind eye to private actions and social institutions that flout the official norm, despite a perceived obligation to defend the norm. In both cases, disadvantaged groups have suffered disproportionately from the current policies, and individuals and groups advocating for reform have encountered multiple roadblocks.

THE CATHOLIC CHURCH AND DIVORCE LAW IN CHILE

During the seventeen years of military dictatorship from 1973 to 1990, the Catholic Church played a progressive role in Chile as the main proponent of respect for human rights and social justice. The church's *Vicaría de Solidaridad* (Vicariate of Solidarity), which defended victims of human rights abuses during the years of the military dictatorship, saved the lives of countless opposition politicians and activists who are now officials in the civilian government and leaders in the center-left government coalition, the *Concertación*. Furthermore, historically the church has been an important wellspring and source of support for efforts to increase socioeconomic justice in Chile. The progressive origins of the Christian Democratic Party, the majority party in the *Concertación*, have their roots in liberation theology movements in the Catholic Church. For these reasons, the church now enjoys a great deal of political influence in Chile, more than in most Latin American countries.[11]

Coincident with this increase in the church's political influence has been the worldwide growth in power of the conservative wing of the church, noted above. The church's increasingly repressive focus on sexual and reproductive rights issues intensified during the 1990s in Chile, strengthening partnerships with the socially conservative opposition parties.[12] The church is thus in the enviable position of having strong alliances with socially conservative politicians of all political tendencies—both from the *Concertación* and from the rightist opposition parties—on policies related to the family, gender, reproduction, and sexuality. As a result, the public discourses in the Congress and in the media regarding proposed legal reforms on issues such as adultery, divorce, same-sex sexual relationships, new reproductive technologies, and abortion are all remarkably uniform in Chile in comparison with other Latin American countries.[13] There is a notable lack of lively public debate on these policies, although most Chileans acknowledge that the private flouting of the policies is widespread. The *doble discurso* is nowhere so amply recognized and commented on as in this socially conservative country.

The countries without a divorce law can be counted on the fingers of one hand, although there is no official United Nations convention that explicitly identifies the right of individuals to separate definitively from their spouses and remarry.[14] The powerful influence of the church on the three civilian governments of the nineties may explain why Chile was one of these countries until 2004. It took fourteen years of legislative efforts to pass the law, although, according to a 1999 survey, 70 percent of Chilean women were in favor of a divorce law.[15] As in most modern industrialized countries, Chilean couples separate and pair up with new partners quite frequently. Many people simply live with a new partner and remain legally separated; others take the precaution of never getting married in the first place. During the 1990s, the courts granted almost 7,000 annulments per year.[16]

Most analysts have recognized that, until 2004, the Chilean legal framework for civilian annulment was a fraudulent safety valve that made up for the absence of a divorce law. The ground most frequently used is that one of the spouses (backed up by two witnesses) swears that she/he gave the wrong address at the time of the wedding ceremony and thus did not fall under the jurisdiction of the official who performed the ceremony.[17] Unfortunately, lawyers' fees make this option unavailable to most low-income people. Certainly one could argue that the lack of the option of divorce resulted in many second unions—especially for low-income families—that were never formalized, thus violating the recognized human right to contract marriage and form a family. One clear result of this situation has been a high and increasing rate of births out of wedlock, which climbed from 30 percent in 1985 to 46 percent in 1999.[18]

An annulment means that legally the marriage never existed, and any division of marital assets is completely up to negotiations between the couple.[19] Therefore, the annulment leaves the custodial parent—usually a woman with fewer assets than her husband and no independent income—without the usual protections regarding rights to assets accumulated during marriage that are incorporated into legal divorces in most countries. Although biological fathers are supposed to pay child support (*pensión alimenticia*), the inefficient justice system cannot guarantee compliance, and so the mothers and children often suffer economically under this arrangement.[20] In this sense, the lack of a divorce law can be argued to constitute discrimination against women, as well as a violation of equality of rights in marriage.[21]

It is clear, then, which social sectors are harmed by the lack of a divorce law. It is less clear why there was so little political will to lead efforts for reform, although there were several attempts. First, it is emotionally and politically possible for Chilean legislators with annulled marriages or legal separations to be vehement opponents of the passage of a divorce law, in the name of the Chilean family and Catholic values. Widespread private transgressions of official norms coexist quite peacefully with public defense of these norms in a double discourse system. Second, the punitive power of the Catholic Church was probably a major factor in the failure of legislative efforts for reform. The church is willing to throw its considerable influence behind successful campaigns to elect socially conservative legislators, and to unseat legislators who lead the efforts to pass divorce laws and other laws expanding sexual and reproductive rights. The label of "*divorcista*" has been attached to reformers.[22]

A divorce law did pass the Chamber of Deputies in 1997, however, thanks to a rare coalition of leaders that included an influential faction within the majority Christian Democratic Party and three legislators from the rightist parties. The bill passed the Chamber with ten votes from rightist parties.[23] At that time, the more conservative Senate defeated the bill. It took seven more years of effort by *Concertación* legislators, and further defections on this issue from the conservative parties, before both bodies in the legislature passed a divorce bill during the government of Ricardo Lagos in 2004. One explanation for this eventual success might be that Lagos is from the Socialist Party, which has fewer ties to the Catholic Church than the previous two *Concertación* governments, led by Christian Democrats. Another is that the determined lobbying by the Catholic Church alienated increasing numbers of legislators from non-*Concertación* parties. However, the Catholic Church persisted and successfully lobbied to weaken the final version, which has a provision that establishes a one-year waiting period for a couple jointly requesting a divorce. If only one partner requests it, the waiting period is three years.

Other legislative developments starting in 1999—such as the passage of a new law abolishing the distinction between legitimate and illegitimate children and a resolution abolishing the law against sodomy—indicate that the political will to act on contentious social issues related to sexuality and reproduction is increasing in Chile.[24]

One factor that may have weakened the political will to push for reform is that professionals with political influence come primarily from middle-class and upper-class backgrounds and could afford the lawyer's fees for an annulment. Although all classes certainly suffered inconveniences and difficulties from the lack of a divorce law, those in a position to affect political decisions did not suffer personally from the most negative consequences of the restrictive legislation.

The lack of strong civilian pressure to pass a divorce law is more puzzling. Even from the women's movement, there was little active pressure on legislators. One feminist legislator who helped lead efforts in the 1990s to push a divorce law through Congress remarked sadly that there were no supporters in the galleries during discussions of the bill. "It seems that [the women's movement] is extremely demobilized, and sometimes I feel very isolated in my efforts," she said.[25]

One study hypothesized that a factor in the relative failure of Chilean feminists to address such issues might be the dispersion of Chilean feminists into NGOs that depend on government contracts for a substantial portion of their income. This dependence would lead to "self-censorship" regarding family law and those sexual and reproductive rights issues that cannot be addressed by the government due to church opposition.[26] Finally, there is widespread recognition, especially among NGOs that engage in community-level work, of the decreased level of mobilization of grassroots women's organizations since the advent of democracy.

As we have seen, the case of divorce law reveals some of the main features of the double discourse system. Because of the escape valves in marriage laws, most of those Chileans who might have had influence on the political process were able to secure an annulment, thus weakening political will for reform. So long as the rule of official silence was respected, political equilibrium was maintained. This equilibrium, however, was also profoundly inequitable toward low-income couples who could not afford annulments and mothers with custody of their children who were not able to negotiate privately a fair settlement regarding marital assets with their spouse.

ABORTION ADVOCACY IN COLOMBIA AND CHILE: WHEN TO BREAK THE SILENCE?

As mentioned in the introduction, there is perhaps no issue related to reproductive rights so hotly contested as the right to safe and legal interruption of unwanted pregnancies.[27] Most reproductive rights advocates hold that this right derives logically from "the right of couples and individuals to decide freely and responsibly the number, spacing and timing of their children."[28] While there are many other arguments in favor of this right, the most widely used are public health and equity arguments, which recognize that the practice of abortions is widespread and that illegality does not stop the practice, but rather drives it underground, causing maternal morbidity and mortality through unsafe abortions, mainly among low-income women.[29] Middle- and upper-income women generally can pay for access to relatively safe clandestine abortion services, but the poor rarely have access to these services. In UN forums and in Catholic countries, public health and equity arguments are gaining ground, but the double discourse system mandates that abortion cannot be officially made legal, even if it is widespread.

El Salvador and Chile share the dubious distinction of being the only countries in the world where all abortions, even to save the mother's life, are illegal and penalized, a legal situation that can be seen to violate the mother's right to life.[30] These laws are even stricter than the Canonical Code of the Catholic Church, which allows abortions in cases of ectopic pregnancies and reproductive cancers.[31] Because of the clandestine nature of induced abortions, the statistics on its prevalence are based on hospital data. The 1994 studies by the Alan Guttmacher Institute (AGI) estimate that there are about 288,400 abortions annually in Colombia and 159,650 in Chile (with total populations of roughly 36 million and 14 million respectively).[32] Other estimates for Colombia range as high as 400,000 per year,[33] and AGI estimated in 1999 that Chile's abortion rate is one of the highest in the world, at 50 per 1,000 births.[34] A nationwide Colombian urban household survey by Lucero Zamudio of the Universidad Externado found that one out of three women who had ever been pregnant had had an abortion.[35] It is estimated that in Chile, 35 of every 100 pregnancies end in abortion, while in Colombia, almost 600 women a year die from complications of abortion, which account for 67 percent of all hospitalizations for gynecological causes.[36] In both countries, mainly low-income women end up in public hospitals due to complications of unsafe abortions. Health providers in the public hospitals who disapprove of abortion often take punishing attitudes toward these patients. There are many accounts not only of hostile remarks, but also of providers performing D&Cs without anesthesia on women with incomplete abortions and forcing women to take medications designed to halt spontaneous abortions.[37]

Nevertheless, in both countries, public opinion regarding abortion is much more progressive than the official policies. A 1997 poll of Colombian women in union (married or in a permanent relationship) found that 20 percent of the respondents had had an abortion, and 48 percent thought that it should be legal under certain circumstances. Much larger majorities thought that abortion should be legal "if the mother was in danger" (88 percent), if the fetus had severe physical or mental defects (78 percent), or in cases of rape (76 percent).[38] The electorate in Chile is perhaps only slightly more conservative on this issue. A 1999 national survey found that high percentages of women favored legal abortion in cases of rape or incest (59 percent), danger to mother's life (78 percent), and fetal problems (70 percent). Fully 30 percent of women thought that abortion should be available "upon the woman's request."[39] These results in Chile are remarkable given the almost complete lack of media coverage of rights-affirming views on abortion.

Despite these similar results, however, the public reactions to the Alan Guttmacher studies in the two countries were startlingly different. There is generally less public debate on the issue of abortion in Chile than in Colombia. In Chile, the publicity surrounding the publication of the Alan Guttmacher statistics was seen to be an intolerable flouting of the *doble discurso* system, according to which infractions are tolerated so long as they remain out of the public view. "*De eso no se habla*" (one doesn't speak of such matters) is the key phrase applied to topics such as abortion. In this case, considerable media coverage and debate following the release of the study in 1994 made the findings impossible to ignore. Although progressive Catholic legislators and officials responded by advocating increased support for family planning services to prevent abortions, conservative legislators revived their attempts to increase the criminal penalties for abortion. In fact, the most tangible result of the publicity was an unusually comprehensive crackdown on clandestine abortion clinics that continued sporadically over the next few years. Even the best-known clinic in the upper-class neighborhood of Providencia was subjected to the police raids. Those who publicized the study did so to point out the futility of penalizing such a widespread practice and the public health consequences of its continued illegality. The consequences of the publicity, however, seem to have been mainly negative and punitive, depriving many women of access to the few safe services that existed.[40]

Colombian society, on the other hand, is less conservative, and the Catholic Church has less influence on public policy there than in Chile. Colombian law provides for legal divorce, freedom of religious instruction in the schools,[41] and mandatory sex education in the schools; the new Health Law 100 guarantees the right to family planning methods. However, in both countries public officials still feel compelled to espouse the Catholic norms, while the church publicly exercises influence to block changes in the abortion laws and to censor AIDS prevention television messages that include condom use.

Abortion services, a few of which operate safely and ethically, are generally much more available in Colombia than in Chile. In the mid-1990s, the author saw full page ads in the daily papers advertising clinics where women could go if they were nervous about "menstrual delays."[42] In addition, many clinics legally provide treatment for incomplete abortions, which are generally started by women in their homes through unsafe methods. Nevertheless, these (or other similar) clinics are raided periodically by the police and shut down. The public reaction to the findings of the Alan Guttmacher study was much more muted in Colombia than in Chile, which may reflect a more widespread knowledge and acceptance of the availability of abortions. The Zamudio study, however, which was released at a regional conference for abortion researchers in Bogotá in November 1994, gained much more media attention, perhaps because the conference itself was a high-profile event attended by legislators from throughout the region. Furthermore, the findings were firmer than the estimates in the Guttmacher study, and therefore less easily ignored. It is not clear whether this media attention was causally linked to a subsequent increase in raids and shutdowns of abortion clinics or whether the raids resulted from other dynamics in the political establishment. At any rate, many of the clinics reopened after a prudent lapse in time.

One Colombian official spoke frankly to the media about how the double discourse system (also called "*doble moral*" or double morality in Colombia) operates with regard to abortion in Colombia: "Abortion is not a problem of legal sanctions, but of collective double morality. There is not a single person who doesn't know where at least one of these medical centers operates, and probably has had occasion to recur to their services. Abortion is an egregious case of clandestine practices that won't disappear."[43]

One explanation for the differences in the level of repression exercised against clandestine providers in the two countries may be the differences in the rule of law. Chile is renowned for its legalistic culture and is known as "the Switzerland of Latin America." Throughout Chilean history, laws and rules in general have been taken very seriously.[44] However, this legalism is selective and arbitrarily applied in the case of laws such as those on abortion that are generally viewed as repressive or as requiring a breach of medical ethics by health providers. For example, in 1994, a significant number of women were in jail in Chile for having undergone an abortion, as documented in a study by lawyer Lidia Casas. However, most of these women were not caught in raids on clinics, but rather denounced by a small minority of health providers.[45] Providers are enjoined by law to denounce women who come to hospitals with complications from induced abortion, thus ostensibly forcing them to breach the confidentiality of the health provider/client relationship. The Casas study, however, suggested that most health providers in Chile respect the confidentiality of this relationship, since the bulk of the denunciations come from a handful of public hospitals serving low-income populations. Furthermore, the denunciations tend to cluster on days when certain doctors are on duty.[46] In this instance, the double discourse system operates by creating a public policy that is privately disregarded, thus saving most women from one of the worst consequences of the policy. However, the unlucky few who fell into the hands of providers who obey the letter of the law were imprisoned. Furthermore, both the risk of mortality/morbidity and the risk of imprisonment fall inequitably on low-income women, who disproportionately end up in public hospitals with complications from unsafe abortions. Middle- and upper-class women, who have access to safer private services, usually escape with impunity. One could argue, as in the case of divorce, that this escape valve weakens the will of political actors in both government and civil society to address this issue in an effective and unified manner.

Colombia, on the other hand, is renowned for widespread impunity for a variety of legal infractions due to its fragile, disorganized, and ineffective system of justice and citizen security/policing.[47] In this country, there is more tolerance for provision of abortion services than in Chile, so long as it remains private and behind-the-scenes, with occasional crackdowns that give a nod to the rule of law and the official discourse condemning abortion. As with other double discourse mechanisms that expand choice, there are no guarantees of accessibility and safety. There seem to be proportionately fewer women who end up in jail in Colombia for abortions than in Chile, although there are no definitive statistics.[48]

The women's and reproductive rights movements in Colombia have suffered from divisions about the best strategy to pursue to decriminalize abortions. Whether the crackdowns that followed the 1994 Zamudio study were coincidental or not, in recent years, nearly every time the issue of abortion has gained prominence in public debates, the repression and crackdowns on clandestine clinics increase, thus incurring negative consequences for women seeking abortions.[49] Thus, there are real advantages in continuing the silence. Furthermore, networks on reproductive rights understand that it is not to their advantage to be solely identified in the public mind with the issue of abortion, which is much more controversial than other sexual and reproductive rights issues in equal need of attention. Similar to legislators, they run political risks if they identify too strongly with this issue.[50]

Unfortunately, another source of division on the issue of abortion in Colombia comes precisely from the efforts of the reproductive rights movement to expand its reach beyond explicitly feminist organizations. This expansion to diverse organizations such as human rights and social justice NGOs and grassroots low-income women's organizations raises the level of disagreement on abortion within the movement. (See Chapter 2.)

Faced with these divisions, the Colombian Sexual and Reproductive Rights Network, which operates in six cities, decided to focus its campaigns in 1997–98 on the issue of sexual violence, in particular on inequities in the laws and the culture and in the judicial treatment of victims. Through this campaign, the network addressed the issue of abortion by advocating for elimination of criminal penalties in cases involving rape. The network had more success in gaining coverage in the local media than in national organs. One could hypothesize that in a double discourse system, the more national (and therefore semi-official) the media outlet, the harder it would be to gain exposure for alternative viewpoints that flout semi-sacred official norms on reproduction and sexuality.

In Chile, the silencing of those who are in favor of depenalizing abortion, or introducing exceptions under which abortion would not be penalized, is much more thorough.[51] Abortion for health reasons or in case of severe fetal defects was legal until 1989, when one of the last acts of the military government was to make it illegal. Yet groups and legislators wishing simply to restore the civil code to its pre-1989 state are vilified in the conservative press. Early in the democratic period, when Congresswoman Adriana Muñoz proposed to restore the clauses allowing therapeutic abortion, she was branded an "abortionist" and defeated on that basis in her reelection campaign in 1993.[52]

In general, socially conservative politicians take the lead on this issue, having introduced repeated initiatives since 1990 to increase the criminal penalties for women who undergo induced abortions. Fortunately, there is just enough awareness in the legislature of the inequitable burden of the criminal penalties for low-income women, and these proposals have all been defeated. Throughout the 1990s and through 2005, progressive legislators and the women's movement have helped to defeat these proposals, although the overall dynamic is still defensive. The Open Forum on Reproductive Rights and Health has been especially active. Formed in 1991, this network of organizations in several provinces has slowly gained more legitimacy. During the 1990s, it was valued by feminists as the only entity within the Chilean women's movement that dared to openly advocate less repressive laws on abortion.[53] Despite this strength, at the time of this study the outreach and effectiveness of the Forum were hampered by several factors. The self-censorship among women's NGOs in Chile in the case of divorce operates even more strongly in the case of abortion advocacy, and so some of the major women's NGOs are not willing to join the Forum or its campaigns. Furthermore, as in Colombia, the Forum encountered diversity of opinion within its ranks on the topic of abortion as their network expanded to provincial cities and to more diverse and grassroots women's organizations. In practice, the network was forced to maintain a policy of voluntary adherence to its campaigns on this issue.

For example, only some regional chapters participate in the Forum's main public strategy on abortion, which is to stand with banners advocating decriminalization of abortion and hand out educational materials in the main city plaza on one Friday of every month. In the tradition of the human rights movement during military dictatorships (most notably the Mothers of the Plaza de Mayo in Argentina), this is a symbolically public statement, bringing a prohibited and ostracized discourse into the most officially public space in the city. It brings citizen disagreement with official policies on taboo topics having to do with reproduction and sexuality out into the open, breaking the logic of the double discourse system. The Forum complemented this strategy, which mainly targets public opinion, with alliances with other NGOs and communications with legislators or government officials when urgent needs for political action arise, as in the case of the 1999 bill that proposed increases in the criminal penalties for abortion.[54] It is puzzling indeed that up until then there was more political activity among Chilean women's NGOs on the much more taboo issue of abortion than on the continuing legislative efforts to pass a divorce law.

The dynamics affecting advocacy for safe and legal abortions in these two countries demonstrate the main features of the double discourse system: the heavy influence of religious dogma on public policy; the violation of women's reproductive rights to voluntary maternity; the existence of informal or illegal mechanisms to expand private choices; the discrimination against low-income women, both in access to these mechanisms and in the arbitrary and haphazard application of punitive laws and practices; divisions within the political class and citizen movements on the issue; and the lack of sufficient political will among both legislators and the women's movement to provide redress.

IMPLICATIONS FOR ADVOCACY: A DISCUSSION

The above examples demonstrate how semi-official, clandestine, and private mechanisms subvert the limitations on exercise of sexual and reproductive rights imposed by repressive policies and deep societal polarization of opinion. One can only applaud human ingenuity in finding so many circuitous ways to expand individual choices in such contexts. The disadvantages of such a system, however, cannot be ignored, because the consequences lead to irreparable harm to so many individuals and families. When solutions that expand sexual and reproductive choices are unofficial, clandestine, and/or dependent on the judgment of professionals such as health providers, no one is guaranteed access to these solutions, no one can oversee their quality, and the health and legal risks fall disproportionately on low-income or marginalized individuals. The informal mechanisms that expand choice generally are safer and more commonly available as one climbs the socioeconomic ladder, thus softening the consequences of repressive policies for members of those very sectors that influence policy decisions, whether from the side of the state or of civil society. This mitigation of consequences combines with the political risks associated with advocacy for sexual and reproductive rights to produce lack of political will to defend these rights. This article has pointed out the risks for legislators; NGOs and those within Catholic institutions also face considerable risks.

Political Costs

Those within Catholic institutions who believe in the principle of freedom of conscience in sexual and reproductive matters suffer disproportionately from repression. The seven organizations in the regional network of Católicas por el Derecho a Decidir (CDD—Catholics for the Right to Decide) have many clandestine supporters who would lose their jobs if they openly declared themselves to be members. The increasing repression of dissident voices within the church has crippled attempts to foster dialogue among the hierarchy; between the hierarchy and clergy (including nuns), who are generally much more flexible and progressive on these issues; and between lay believers and the hierarchy. Several brave clergy who have voiced their pro-rights views in publications and in the media have been "silenced," with well-known examples in Colombia and Brazil.[55] In 1999, a prominent researcher in the physiology of reproduction from the Catholic University in Chile lost his professorship when he published an article in the newspaper *El Mercurio* using arguments from Catholic theology to oppose the Larrain bill, which would have increased criminal penalties for abortion.[56] In the face of this repression, Catholics for Free Choice and the Latin American partner network Católicas por el Derecho a Decidir (CDD) have used research (for example, publishing results of focus groups of Catholic women on these issues) and public opinion polls. In 2004, surveys of Catholics in Bolivia, Colombia, and Mexico demonstrated the mismatch between the private reality and opinions of lay Catholics and the public discourse of the hierarchy.[57] Through publications and speaking tours, CDDs in seven countries have also publicized the views of dissident Catholic theologians to legitimate their point of view. Unfortunately, the Catholic Church is not a democracy, and these strategies have less power to sway church leaders than they would when used by lay advocates to influence elected legislators. Nevertheless, such research and media exposure still serves a key purpose by helping to legitimize a pro-rights discourse in countries whose public policies are heavily influenced by the church.

Citizen advocacy groups, many of whom are women's NGOs, are often unable to be as persistent and as effective as antirights activists are. In the cases cited above in Chile and Colombia, citizen activists did not mobilize sufficiently on these issues for a variety of political, economic, and cultural reasons. On the economic side, due to dramatic decreases in foreign aid, many Latin American NGOs have been suffering from such a precarious financial situation that their ability to be a consistent and independent voice in public debates is in peril. Not only are the few remaining staff completely overextended, but also the NGOs are in such precarious situations that it is a big risk to make an organizational decision to carry the banner for controversial issues. Lacking foreign aid and private national donors for often-controversial programs, the NGOs have begun to depend on local and national government contracts, or on bilateral and multilateral contracts that must be approved by governments, for a significant portion of their funding. In several cases in the region, opposing the government's official position on sexual and reproductive rights issues has made an NGO persona non grata with government agencies. As a result, the NGO is unofficially excluded from winning government contracts or consulting jobs, no matter how unrelated to the NGO's stand on sexual and reproductive rights.

Possible Strategies

An analysis of the logic of the double discourse system suggests three possible strategies to increase the political will for change: using both public health and ethical arguments, decreasing the political risks for various political actors, and eliminating the safety valves. The latter path would be greatly mistaken and would only increase suffering and harm. It would produce the same effects as the Chilean crackdowns on illegal abortion providers, narrowing the choices for thousands of desperate women and couples and probably leading them to take more unsafe measures to end their pregnancies.[58] The safety valves exist because there is a demand for them that will not be denied, no matter what the official policies.

How then can advocacy strategies address the double discourse system? On issues from divorce to abortion, the main strategies have been to point out the obvious epidemiological facts in lobbying efforts: adolescents are sexually active, women are having abortions, mothers are dying, and couples are separating. Armed with information on the negative consequences for public health of rights-denying policies, advocates lobby behind the scenes and in professional conferences to sway policymakers.

In all advocacy strategies, it is important to study one's audience and to tailor approaches to diverse groups within the ranks. There is a more or less hidden diversity within the corps of legislators and public officials on these issues in most countries. The most vehement defenders of rights, on the one hand, and of semisacred norms limiting rights, on the other, are only the most visible and obvious audiences. Using audience analysis, there is a key flaw in the strategy that depends on public health and equity arguments with regard to the subset of legislators who strongly defend limits to rights on religious grounds: the epidemiological facts will not sway someone who is defending a sacred norm. In Christian religious thinking, the fact that people transgress or sin does not mean that the Ten Commandments should be thrown out the window. In this view, suffering because of transgression does not constitute an injustice. Morality is conflated with the law, and so making divorce, abortion, or adultery legal is tantamount to giving these acts moral approval.

Besides the public health and equity arguments, there is another argument that may be more effective with these most intransigent opponents of sexual and reproductive rights, and more compelling to believers in all religions: the principle of religious diversity. A group of religious leaders from all of the world's major religions, including a representative from the socially conservative sector of the Catholic Church hierarchy, was convened before the ICPD to discuss reproductive rights issues. A key principle that they all agreed on was that no religion should have the power, through the state or by other means, to impose its precepts on the believers of any other religion. Religious diversity has increased significantly in Latin America and in most traditionally Catholic countries, making this an important argument for advocates.[59] One complementary advocacy strategy would thus be to forge alliances with believers in religions other than Catholicism to demand that state policies not be linked to the doctrines of any one religion.[60]

Advocates of sexual and reproductive rights do not face arguments based only in religious doctrine. Increasingly, opponents of reform are also using the discourse of human rights, citing the fetus's right to life, or the parents' right to control the education of their adolescent children. Unfortunately, this type of argument falsely pits rights against rights, resulting in stalemated discussions: adolescents' rights against those of parents, and women's rights against those of fetuses. In Latin America, however, the Catholic doctrines of human life and rights beginning at conception and the inadmissibility of premarital sex are embedded in these arguments, so that it is useful for sexual and reproductive rights advocates to deconstruct them to show their basis in one dominant religion's doctrines.

While it is important to understand the belief system of the most committed opponents of sexual and reproductive rights, the use of public health information and equity arguments is still an effective strategy with other policymakers who may be more open to perspectives based on the right to health. This discussion will focus on two less visible audiences present in many legislatures and government agencies: (1) those who have not given the issues much attention and take the traditional stance as the path of least resistance, and (2) those who are already in favor of sexual and reproductive rights but voice these opinions only behind the scenes.

The first audience may not have seriously examined the issues or may have little information; being politicians, they have taken the safe road, which is usually to espouse the traditional norms. This group may be more open to persuasion by information on the inequitable and public health consequences of repressive laws and norms, especially if public opinion seems to be leaning in the direction of reform. One advocate discussed this group as follows:

Lack of information plays an important role among decision-makers with regard to reproductive issues in many countries. I have interviewed legislators who have no idea of the implications of passing restrictive laws and have never heard different points of view on abortion. ... The Catholic Church steps into this information vacuum, bringing their lobbyists to the Congress with sensationalist videos on abortion. Unfortunately, the women's groups don't have the same capacity for reaction and mobilization in any [Latin American] countries.[61]

This quotation illustrates the importance of the media in airing diverse points of view and the imbalance in the mobilizing capacity between antirights and pro-rights lobbyists.

The second audience consists of those legislators and public officials who take rights-affirming stances on sexual and reproductive health issues in private. There are fierce behind-the-scenes disagreements within governmental agencies, political parties, and committees, too often resulting in bland and meaningless consensus statements, or simply in inaction. Anecdotes about these controversies in private conversations are as common as weeds, but how rare it is that such disagreements come into the public light so that the citizenry can somehow weigh into the debate! Within most agencies and political parties, maintaining the appearance of public consensus is an unquestioned value. As a result, the "legitimate" discourse with guaranteed access to the media is still that of the Catholic Church hierarchies or public figures who agree with them, while the proactive voices in defense of sexual and reproductive rights rarely reach the public eye and ear except when the church is attacking them. This dynamic accords unequal footing to pro-rights discourses in policy debates, perpetuates the political marginalization of rights advocates, and keeps disagreements among political actors safely behind the scenes.

As long as the political costs of espousing controversial pro-rights proposals remain so high, the most effective short-term political strategy for advocates is to obey the logic of the double discourse system by conducting negotiations and lobbying behind the scenes, out of the public eye. In both Colombia and Chile, most current advocacy efforts for abortion law reform are low-key and effectively out of sight. Advocates defend this strategy on ethical grounds, because public debates have resulted in increased repression. This strategy might result in some legal gains, but in the long term it fails to solve the problem of the perceived illegitimacy and immorality of pro-rights stances on these controversial issues in the public realm.

How can the political culture be changed so that bringing these debates into the public view is less costly, both for the advocates and for the men and women who most suffer from the double discourse system? How can the defensive dynamic be turned around, so that the pro-rights forces could play a proactive role in national debates, rather than responding to initiatives that would erode rights even further? It is clear that various advocacy strategies must focus on reducing political risks for potential advocates. One common strategy is to increase the presence of rights-affirming voices in the mass media, bringing hitherto private opinions into the open. Increased exposure to the arguments on both sides helps to legitimize the debate itself as well as pro-rights positions, and to reduce the political costs of engaging in debate and taking such positions publicly.

With the same aim, many reproductive rights advocacy groups have used public opinion surveys to legitimize rights perspectives. Surveys can help to persuade politicians that defending rights is consistent with the views of their constituents and thus might come with fewer political costs than they fear.[62] Complementing such surveys with those of Catholics conducted by CDD might be doubly effective in showing politicians the extent of the distance between their constituents and the hierarchy within the church.

As mentioned above, in both Colombia and Chile, one of the sources of division within the women's movement on abortion has been precisely their effort to broaden their social base by including more grassroots and low-income women's organizations. Broadening the coalition that is pro-rights, however, is indeed a promising strategy for civil society groups. The more diverse and broad-based the groups that are supporting rights, the lower the political risk of defending those rights. Although such organizations are much more apt to be ideologically diverse than the feminist NGOs, it is precisely these low-income sectors that suffer the brunt of the negative consequences of rights-denying policies and have the most to gain from policy reform. Therefore, it would be advantageous to create partnerships with subgroups within these organizations, if not with the organization as a whole.

Finally, many women's organizations and pro-rights public officials have followed the strategy of using the consensus documents and conventions signed by the leaders of their country to monitor the country's progress toward the implementation of the accords or treaties. Although the Programme of Action from the ICPD and the Platform for Action from the Fourth World Conference on Women in Beijing reflect compromises on some sexual and reproductive rights issues, notably on the issue of the right to access to safe abortion, their recommendations have still proved to be invaluable instruments for advocacy to expand access to safe, abortion where it is legal. Some women's NGOs use the reporting process to the CEDAW Committee as an important opportunity at national level to work with governments—or through the mechanism of shadow reports (to collect and analyze information on the status of women's rights—including sexual and reproductive rights) within their countries. On the other hand, at least in some countries in Latin America, the reporting process for the Committee on the Rights of the Child is a relatively under-used resource for advocates of adolescent sexual and reproductive health policies and programs. The concluding comments and observations of the treaty bodies on these issues are excellent tools for advocacy. This strategy is so useful precisely because it legitimates sexual and reproductive health and rights as global human rights under international law, thus reducing the political risks of advocacy.

For all potential advocates of sexual and reproductive rights, whether in government, civil society, or the church, the political risks of publicly defending these rights are probably the key obstacle to attaining a critical mass of supporters. It is one thing to agree privately that sexual and reproductive choices should be a matter of personal conscience rather than law and to avail oneself privately of all of the mechanisms to expand such choices. It is a completely different thing to take on the political costs associated with committing oneself wholeheartedly to advocacy on behalf of controversial issues such as depenalization of abortion.

Before designing strategies, an important exercise for advocates is to analyze the nature of the risks, as well as the sources, the arguments, and the tactics of attacks. Multifaceted strategies that use a combination of tactics to reduce these risks and effectively counter attacks—for example, public opinion polls, alliances on other issues, international agreements, partnerships with media, and education of policymakers—are most effective, because such tactics are mutually reinforcing. Analyzing the differences among potential allies is also important in order to approach each of them appropriately.

As modern societies become ever more diverse in belief systems and in cultural or religious traditions, undue influence of one religious doctrine on the state will become less and less acceptable. The blurring of the distinction between what is considered immoral and what should be illegal greatly hampers efforts in Latin America to protect sexual and reproductive rights. Acceptance of diversity of opinions and belief systems among citizens of a country, and indeed among the believers in any religion, is one cornerstone of democracy, and of the defense of sexual and reproductive rights. Respect for human rights is the other. Sexuality and reproduction are key aspects of human life and welfare, in relation to which governments should be held accountable to their obligation to promote comprehensive physical, emotional, and social health and well-being.

NOTES

1. This chapter is reprinted with some updates and changes with the kind permission of the journal *Health and Human Rights,* published by the François-Xavier Bagnoud Center for Health and Human Rights, Harvard School of Public Health, Volume 4, No 2, 2000. For the most part, the descriptions of policies and the situation of NGOs correspond to the situation at the time the article was written in 1999, but updates from 2004–2005 reflect the passage of a divorce law in Chile in 2004.

2. Programme of Action of the International Conference on Population and Development, Report of the International Conference on Population and Development, September 5–13, 1994, UN Doc. A/CONF.171/13, para. 7.3. The reservations expressed by Argentina in the "Cairo+5" meetings in 1999 coordinated by UNFPA represent an exception to the general consensus in Latin America.

3. Belden, Russonello & Stewart, *Attitudes of Catholics on Reproductive Rights, Church-State, and Related Issues,* Washington, DC: Catholics for Free Choice and Católicas por el Derecho a Decidir en Bolivia, Colombia y Mexico, 2003; Catholics for Free Choice, *Catholics and Reproduction: A World View,* Washington, DC: CFFC, 1994.

4. L. Haas, "The Catholic Church in Chile," in C. Smith and J. Prokopy (eds.), *Latin American Religion in Motion,* New York and London: Routledge, 1999; Mala Htun, "Church and State in the Struggle for Divorce," Chapter 4 in M. Htun (ed.), *Sex and the State: Divorce, and the Family Under Latin American Dictatorships and Democracies,* Cambridge, UK: Cambridge University Press, 2003. See also M. Blofield, "The Politics of Abortion in Chilean and Argentina: Public Opinion, Social Actors and Discourse, and Political Agendas," presented at Latin American Studies Association conference, Chicago, September 1998.

5. R. Petchesky, and K. Judd (eds.) for the International Reproductive Rights Action Group (IRRRAG), *Negotiating Reproductive Rights,* New York: Zed Books, 1998, 17.

6. The author worked in these countries from 1992 to 1998 as the program officer in charge of the Ford Foundation's Sexual and Reproductive Health Program, based in the Andean Region and Southern Cone office in Santiago, Chile.

7. I am indebted to Mari Luz Silva, one of the designers of the Chilean government's sex education program, for serving as the original inspiration for this article with her thoughts on Catholic cultures and the double discourse.

8. The Philippines is the main example outside of Latin America of a state heavily influenced by Catholicism. It would be interesting to analyze whether the double discourse system operates in countries with other hegemonic religions as well.

9. From the author's conversations with members of Católicas por el Derecho a Decidir network in six Latin American countries.

10. Koinonia [organization of theologians], *Problemática Religiosa de la Mujer que Aborta,* Bogotá, Colombia: Universidad Externado de Colombia, 1996. Also presented at a World Health Organization meeting of Latin American researchers on abortion at the Universidad Externado de Colombia, Bogotá, Colombia, November 1994.

11. L. Haas, "The Catholic Church in Chile," in C. Smith and J. Prokopy (eds.) (1999), 60 describes how church officials "collect the bill" (*cobran la cuenta*) in their lobbying of representatives of the Left who received protection from the church.

12. John Paul II's conservative appointments of bishops started during the military dictatorship, strengthening the faction of the church that was allied with the military government even as progressive sectors of the church led the efforts to protect human rights. See L. Haas 1999 op. cit. and M. Htun 2003 for a full discussion.

13. The ownership of Chilean newspapers and television stations is concentrated in two large conglomerates and the Catholic Church, all of which tend to have socially

conservative editorial policies. See M. Blofield, 22, op. cit. (see note 4); Uca Silva of Sur Profesionales, Santiago, also analyzes the effect on public debates of this concentration in an unpublished 1996 report to the Ford Foundation's Andean and Southern Cone office.

14. Until 2004, Chile, Malta, and Andorra were the only countries with no divorce law. The Universal Declaration of Human Rights, G.A. Res. 217A (III), UN GAOR, Res. 71, UN Doc. A/810 (1948), Art. 16.1 states that "Men and women of full age, without any limitation due to race, nationality or religion, have the right to marry and to found a family. They are entitled to equal rights as to marriage, during marriage and at its dissolution," thus implicitly recognizing dissolution as part of the right to marriage. Articles 23.2 and 23.4 of the International Covenant on Civil and Political Rights, G. A. Res. 2200 (XXI), UN GAOR, 21st Sess., Supp. No. 16, at 49, UN Doc. A/6316 (1966) contain similar language. Applying the logic of implicit recognition, the most recent report of the UN Committee on Human Rights on Chile (CCPR/C/79/Add.104, para. 17) said that the lack of a divorce law might constitute a violation of Article 23. Thanks to Luisa Cabal of the Center for Reproductive Rights and Gaby Oré Aguilar for thoughts and references.

15. Grupo Iniciativa Mujeres, "Encuesta Nacional: Opinión y Actitudes de las Mujeres Chilenas sobre la Condición de Género," January 1999, carried out by Quanta Sociología Aplicada, using a nationally representative urban sample of 1,800 women in 22 cities. For an excellent in-depth analysis of the issue of divorce in Chile, see Chapter 4 in M. Htun, "Church and State in the Struggle for Divorce," 2003.

16. M. Aylwin and I. Walker, *The Chilean Family: Aspirations, Realities, and Challenges,* 1996, 121, quoted in M. Htun 2003.

17. This provision has its basis in canon law, in which it was assumed priests would know the situation of couples residing in the same neighborhood well enough to prevent them from being married if there were important impediments, such as too close a relation or an existing spouse. The opinion in the Supreme Court case of Sabioncello con Haussman (March 28, 1932) reads: "It is legitimate to prove the lack of competence of the Official of the Civil Registry by means of the witnesses' testimony [that neither of the spouses lived within the jurisdiction of that official] during the annulment proceedings." Quoted in H. Corral, "Iniciativas Legales sobre Familia y Divorcio," in *Controversia sobre Familia y Divorcio,* Santiago: Ediciones Universidad Católica de Chile, 1997, 172.

18. This high rate is explained by both nonformalized unions and adolescent pregnancies. A new law giving children born inside and outside of marriage equal rights and benefits took effect in 1999; see C. Gutierrez, "46% de niños chilenos nacen fuera del matrimonio," [46 percent of Chilean children are born outside of marriage] October 27, 1999, *La Tercera* [newspaper].

19. M. Htun 2003.

20. Instituto de la Mujer in Chile, unpublished 1996 research report on "Food pensions."

21. As established in Article 23.2.4 of the ICCPR (see note 14).

22. There is definitely less stigma attached to advocating for a divorce law, however, than for a law on "therapeutic" abortion, which in current debates in Chile would include legality of abortion in cases of rape, incest, and severe fetal anomalies.

23. L. Haas (1999), 60, and M. Htun 2003, Chapter 4. Htun provides an in-depth analysis of the "reformist coalitions" promoting divorce in the 1990s and of the dynamics within the corps of Christian Democrat legislators.

24. See C. Kraus, "Victoria Would Not Be Amazed by Chile Today," October 24, 1999, *New York Times.* Haas 1999 also agrees with this assessment, quoting several rightist deputies to document her perception that members of the political right are defecting from their formerly uniform support for the church's lobbying efforts.

25. María Antonieta Saa, deputy to the Congress, quoted in an unpublished 1997 study by Peruvian sociologist Maruja Barrig, "De Cal y Arena: ONGs y Movimiento de Mujeres en Chile," 17.

26. M. Barrig 1997, 16.

27. The main sources for this section on Colombia and Chile are the NGO shadow reports for the 20th session of the CEDAW Committee for both countries. Both are available in English and Spanish. For Colombia, see Center for Reproductive Rights (then called Center for Reproductive Law and Policy—CRLP) and Corporación Casa de la Mujer, *Derechos Reproductivos de la Mujer en Colombia: Un Reporte Sombra,* New York and Bogotá: CRLP and Corporación Casa de la Mujer, 1998; The Chilean NGO shadow report, *The Rights of Women in Chile* New York and Santiago, 1999, was cowritten by CRLP, the Comité Latinoamericano y del Caribe para la Defensa de los Derechos de la Mujer (CLADEM), Foro Abierto de Salud y Derechos Sexuales y Reproductivos, and Corporación de la Mujer, La Morada.

28. ICPD Programme of Action (see note 1), para. 7.3.

29. Although hospital data on abortion are widely acknowledged to be under-reported, in the mid-1990s abortion still figured in official data as the first cause of maternal mortality in seven Latin American Countries, including Chile; see FLACSO (Chile) and Instituto de la Mujer (Spain), *Mujeres Latinoamericanas en Cifras: Tomo Comparativo,* Santiago, Chile: FLACSO, 1995, 131.

30. The map of countries and restrictions is available from the Center for Reproductive Rights, accessed on November 1, 2005: http://www.reproductiverights.org/pub_fac_abortion_laws.html. In most lists, Colombia is counted as a country allowing abortion in cases of threat to the woman's life or physical health, but in fact the law is ambiguous. No. 5, Article 29 in the Colombian Penal Code can be interpreted as depenalizing interruptions of pregnancy in "estado de necesidad" (state of necessity) to protect the life or health of the mother. Protection in these cases is open to interpretation by individual judges and thus is not guaranteed. For a full discussion of the legal situation of abortion in Colombia, see D. Arcila, "El Aborto Voluntario en Colombia: Urgencia de un Abordaje Jurídico Integral," in *Perspectivas en Salud y Derechos Sexuales y Reproductivos,* Medellín, Colombia: CERFAMI, 1999, 14–22.

31. Personal communication from Dr. José Barzelatto, Center for Health and Social Policy.

32. Alan Guttmacher Institute. *An Overview of Clandestine Abortion in Latin America,* New York: Alan Guttmacher Institute, 1996.

33. "Aborto: Informe Especial," *Cambio 16,* February 1997, 20–23, quoted in D. Arcila 1999.

34. "Induced Abortion Worldwide," Facts in Brief, Alan Guttmacher Institute, from a 1999 publication, accessed on November 1, 2005: http://www.guttmacher.org/pubs/fb_0599.html#13.

35. L. Zamudio, presentations to the Meeting of Researchers on Induced Abortion in Latin America and the Caribbean at the Universidad Externado, Bogotá, November 1994, and the Latin American and Caribbean Parliamentarians' Meeting on Abortion, Bogotá, October 1998.

36. Arcila 1999, 8, op. cit. (see note 30).

37. D&C stands for dilation and curettage—that is, the scraping of all remains of the fetus from the uterus in cases of incomplete abortion. The account of forced medication comes from a conversation with the Medellín, Colombia chapter of the National Network for Sexual and Reproductive Rights in the mid-1990s. In the author's experience, anecdotes about hostile remarks are almost universal when talking with researchers and activists who work with the health sector and community groups on the issue of abortion.

38. January 29, 1997 survey by the Centro Nacional de Consultoría, quoted in Arcila 1999, 22, op. cit. (see note 30).

39. See Grupo Iniciativa Mujeres 1999, op. cit. (note 15).

40. I was first alerted to this issue in a conversation with anthropologist Monica Weisner, the researcher for the Alan Guttmacher study. Most informants in the Chilean women's movement believe that safe clandestine abortion services became scarcer after 1994 than they were previously, and now the clandestine referral networks often have no referrals to offer. At last inquiry in December 2004, the cost of a safe surgical legal abortion in Chile varied from US$1,000 to $1,500. The minimum wage in 2004 is approximately US$200 a month, and the median monthly family wage is US$660.

41. In Chile, the author's personal experience shows that a course on Catholic religion is mandatory in all schools, public and private, and can only be taught by instructors certified by a Catholic institute. Parents of children of other faiths must request to be excused from the class and cannot organize an alternative class on, say, world religions.

42. Examples of these ads can also be found in the article "Aborto: ¿Hora de legalizar" Semana, February 9–16, 1993, 41.

43. Ibid.

44. The glaring exception to this trend has been the amnesty for the human rights abuses committed during the dictatorship. This amnesty is now, however, subject to serious legal challenges both within Chile and from abroad.

45. Lidia Casas, Women Behind Bars, New York: Center for Reproductive Law and Policy, and Santiago: Open Forum on Reproductive Health and Rights, 1998. A Spanish language edition is also available. Recent inquiries with police authorities in 2003 by the Católicas por el Derecho a Decidir organization in Chile suggest that women who are denounced for induced abortions are no longer sent to jail in Chile.

46. Personal communication from José Barzelatto.

47. Ninety-eight percent of all court cases do not result in a sentence. In cases of homicide, 95 percent of the cases are never solved; source: Mauricio Rubio, Crimen sin sumario. Análisis Geoeconómico de la Justicia Colombiana, Bogotá: Centro de Estudios para el Desarrollo de la Universidad de los Andes, 1996. The Consejo

Superior de Judicatura disputes this figure and estimates impunity at 60 percent, which is still extremely high. Personal communication from Carmen Posada, lawyer and executive director of CERFAMI (Center of Integrated Resources for Families) in Medellín.

48. In 1991, there were 137 court cases and 29 people imprisoned for abortion in Colombia; see "Aborto: ¿Hora de legalizar" (note 42). In comparison, the Chilean study (Casas 1998, op. cit. note 45) shows that 57 percent of the women who had abortions and whose cases were reviewed spent time in prison, and 36 percent were held for more than two weeks. The study also reports that 22 women in the small provincial city of Puerto Montt were in jail for abortion at the time of a visit by the Open Forum, a reproductive health NGO network. Given that Colombia has 2.6 times the population of Chile, the level of repression in Chile is clearly much higher. With the high levels of impunity for other crimes in Colombia, however, it is telling that so many women end up in jail for abortion.

49. Many personal communications from Colombian colleagues over the years, most recently from Carmen Posada.

50. See full discussion of this issue in Chapter 2.

51. Current proposals would allow abortion to save the woman's life and health or in cases of severe fetal defects or rape and incest, under the misnomer of "therapeutic abortion."

52. She regained her seat in the next elections in 1997, however, Mala Htun (personal communication) notes that other sponsors of the bill were not defeated. It would be interesting to analyze what circumstances made her more vulnerable.

53. M. Barrig 1997. The situation has changed since the Barrig study; there are other organizations involved in abortion advocacy in Chile in 2004–2005.

54. This was known as the Larrain bill. Personal communication from Josefina Hurtado of the Forum, October 1999.

55. The best-known example from Brazil is that of Sister Yvone Gerbara, who gave an interview to the national magazine *Veja* in which she advocated depenalization of abortion. In Colombia, Alberto Munera, a prominent Jesuit theologian, was deprived of his teaching post in 1995 after he defended ICPD principles on a national television program.

56. This was Dr. Horacio Croxatto from the Instituto Chileno de Medicina Reproductiva (ICMER). Personal communications from Dr. José Barzelatto and several other Chilean colleagues.

57. Belden, Russonello & Stewart. 2003, op. cit.

58. It would be important to conduct a follow-up study in Chile to the 1994 Guttmacher study to verify whether in fact there are fewer providers than before, although an important confounding factor is that medication abortion has become more widely available since that study was done.

59. I am indebted to Dr. José Barzelatto for consistently pointing out the importance of this agreement; see "World Religions and the 1994 UN International Conference on Population and Development: A Report on an International and Interfaith Consultation," Chicago, IL: Park Ridge Center for the Study of Health, Faith, and Ethics, 1994. For a full discussion of increased religious diversity in Latin America, see C. Smith and J. Prokopy 1999.

60. According to the 1992 census, about 13.4 percent of the Chilean population are Evangelical/Protestant, while 76.7 percent are Catholic. Atheists make up 5.8 percent of the population, and "other religions" (probably mainly Jewish and Muslim) make up 4.24 percent; see F. Kamsteeg, "Pentecostalism and Political Awakening in Pinochet's Chile and Beyond," in C. Smith and J. Prokopy 1999. More recent studies show an increase in the percentage of Evangelicals to 16 percent and a decrease in the percentage of Catholics to 72 percent; see *Diario El Segundo,* December 17, 1998, quoted in a personal communication from Josefina Hurtado.

61. Personal communication from Luisa Cabal, staff attorney, Center for Reproductive Rights.

62. Besides CDDs in Mexico, Colombia, and Bolivia, other groups include Calandria, a communications NGO in Peru, as well as Grupo Impulsora in Peru and Grupo Iniciativa in Chile—two post–Beijing NGO networks.

2

NGO ADVOCACY NETWORKS IN LATIN AMERICA: LESSONS FROM EXPERIENCE IN PROMOTING WOMEN'S AND REPRODUCTIVE RIGHTS

Networks entangle us, but they have opened many doors.[1]

INTRODUCTION

This chapter analyzes the experiences during the 1990s[2] of thirteen Latin American regional and national networks[3] of nongovernmental organizations (NGOs) that advocate for the issues of sexual and reproductive rights and women's rights. Although the chapter includes some observations on regional NGO advocacy networks, its primary focus is on national networks.

Research for this study addressed three interlocking questions:

1. What tensions arise when NGO networks strive to become political actors in the national and regional arenas, and how does their internal governance affect their ability to handle such tensions constructively?

This chapter is reprinted with some changes and updates with the permission of the North-South Center Press at the University of Miami; *NGO Advocacy Networks in Latin America: Lessons from Experience in Promoting Women's and Reproductive Rights in Latin America* was published previously as North-South Agenda Paper #61 of The Dante B. Fascell North-South Center at the University of Miami, 2003; a shorter Spanish version based on an earlier draft of this article was published as "Redes de ONGs reivindicativas en América Latina: Lecciones de la experiencia de promover los derechos reproductivos y de la mujer," in *La Salud como Derecho Ciudadano—Perspectivas y Propuestas desde America Latina*, edited by Carlos Cáceres, M. Cueto, M. Ramos, S. Vallenas, conference proceedings of the VI Congreso Latinoamericano de Ciencias Sociales y Salud, Lima, Peru: Universidad Peruana Cayetano Heredia, 2001.

2. What factors enable or pose obstacles to the political advocacy of these networks?

3. Given the above factors, what strategies are the NGO advocacy networks best suited to pursue, and what other strategies are best left to other configurations of social actors?

The learning curve for the newer national networks has been steep, with many common elements, yet there has been little communication among networks about what they have learned. In this age of globalization and global policy processes, new networks emerge all the time and could benefit from the experience of the existing Latin American networks. This chapter aims to present what the NGO networks in this study have learned about how to face common advocacy challenges.

This study and the networks in it define *advocacy* in its broadest sense, that is, to "include all strategies and actions designed to promote the implementation or reform of legal frameworks and policies, and to stimulate civil society's participation in these political processes. Therefore, these advocacy strategies address not only the political system, but also the cultural, social, and economic structures affecting a certain group. In this broad approach, participants and audiences include governments, other social actors, and the general public."[4] The implication of this approach to advocacy is that the strategies employed by advocacy NGOs and their networks are multifaceted and vary enormously.

My interest in studying NGO advocacy networks stems from the participant-observer role I had as a representative of international agencies that supported these networks, first in the Women's Programs Division of The Pathfinder Fund[5] in the 1980s, and then as program officer in charge of the Sexual and Reproductive Health Program for the Ford Foundation's Andean and Southern Cone office in Santiago, Chile, between 1992 and 1998. At the Ford Foundation, support for NGO networks was the linchpin of our program strategy to strengthen advocacy efforts for sexual and reproductive rights and women's rights in the region. Therefore, I was intimately involved during the 1990s in the initial stages of country networks in Chile, Peru, and Colombia and throughout the 1980s and 1990s in the formative moments of some regional networks. In addition to these personal experiences, this study draws on data from project evaluations, internal documents, and in-depth individual and group interviews conducted in Chile, Peru, Colombia, and Mexico from October 1998 through February 2000.[6]

The support of NGO advocacy networks by the Ford Foundation and other donors is based on the belief that networks strengthen advocacy efforts in several ways:

- NGO members of networks can complement each other's efforts through diversity in areas of expertise and in access to key audiences such as public officials, religious leaders, and the mass media. Their diversity can allow a division of labor and synergy of efforts, with all members working toward the same broad goals but with different tactics and/or in different arenas.

- Having a large number of organizations speak with a united voice in policy debates can increase the legitimacy of pro-rights stances and, thus, the chances that the advocates' views will carry more weight.
- NGO networks hold the promise of breaking down inequalities and isolation between groups in national capitals and in provinces,[7] thus addressing the needs and concerns of the relatively underprivileged and isolated provincial groups.
- Sharing information and learning from experience can prevent smaller and newer groups from repeating mistakes and having to reinvent the wheel.
- National networks can function as an efficient link between national groups and international networks and policy processes.

Many funding agencies share other administrative, programmatic, and pragmatic reasons for supporting NGO networks. First, most agencies strive to keep their administrative costs under control by limiting the number of grant actions, and program officers are under pressure to limit the number of small grants.[8] A substantial grant to an NGO network can benefit a large number of smaller groups, directly or indirectly, at the same administrative cost as a small grant to one group. With a network grant, a program officer who does not have the time to travel to provinces or the ability to make small grants can still provide benefit to the relatively underprivileged groups in the provinces. In addition, program officers view grants to networks as a way of providing an incentive for collaboration, instead of competition, among NGOs. Finally, program officers (especially those based in countries outside that of the grant in question) may feel that they have neither enough information nor the time to acquire enough information to make sound choices among NGOs competing for funds. Given all these programmatic and donor-driven reasons for investments in networks, it is paradoxical that NGO networks often face such difficulties in raising funds. This study will examine some of the reasons for these difficulties.

The formation of new NGO networks in the 1990s was favored by the tremendous policy successes of transnational civil society networks during the 1990s at the UN conferences on human rights, the environment, population, and women's rights.[9] The following brief summary of this recent history surrounding the international successes of NGO networks helps explain the origins of the national NGO networks on women's rights and reproductive rights in this study and the high hopes surrounding them.

LATIN AMERICAN NGO ADVOCACY NETWORKS FOR WOMEN'S RIGHTS AND SEXUAL AND REPRODUCTIVE RIGHTS: HISTORY AND CONTEXT

Margaret E. Keck and Kathryn Sikkink have analyzed the civil society advocacy networks that emerged in tandem with social movements for human rights, women's rights, and the environment in the 1980s and 1990s.

They described the close relationship of the transnational women's advocacy networks to the UN conferences as follows:

The emergence of international women's networks was more intertwined with the UN system than the other networks [human rights, environmental] discussed in this book. Chronologies of the international women's movement are largely a litany of UN meetings. ... International conferences did not create women's networks, but they legitimized the issues and brought together unprecedented numbers of women from around the world. Such face-to-face encounters generate the trust, information sharing, and discovery of common concerns that [give] impetus to network formation.[10]

In Latin America, the first networks on women's rights were informal efforts of individual feminists, arising from preparations for the First World Conference on Women in 1975 and then from continued networking after that conference during the UN Decade for Women (1976–1985). The first Latin American Feminist Meeting (Encuentro Feminista) was held in 1981, and the meetings continue to this day, operating more within a "logic of mutual solidarity and identity" than within a "logic of transnational advocacy,"[11] In 1984, at a meeting in Tensa, Colombia, supported by several U.S. and European agencies, the participants founded the Latin American and Caribbean Women's Health Network (LACWHN).

In 1985, the Third World Conference on Women in Nairobi witnessed an enormous increase in representation of women around the world in the NGO Forum,[12] and it provided the occasion for the formation of three regional networks focused on women and rights, of which one was the Latin American and Caribbean Committee for the Defense of Women's Rights (Comité de América Latina y el Caribe para la Defensa de los Derechos de la Mujer—CLADEM).

The decade of the 1990s witnessed the formation of a diverse range of new national and regional networks, spurred by unprecedented NGO involvement and donor funding for that involvement in national, regional, and global consultation processes for four major issue-oriented United Nations conferences: Environment in Rio de Janeiro (1992); Human Rights in Vienna (1993); Population and Development (ICPD) in Cairo (1994); and Fourth World Conference on Women (FWCW) in Beijing (1995).[13] At the same time, advocacy networks of HIV/AIDS activists organized from global to local levels in response to the onset of the HIV/ AIDS epidemic, linking health to human rights issues in a series of UN-sponsored global meetings. Following these impressive global policy achievements of civil society advocacy networks during the 1990s, the challenge for NGO networks has been to translate these important policy gains in international UN consensus documents into national policies and programs.

In Latin America, as in other regions, new national advocacy networks were formed as part of national consultation processes leading up to the

UN conferences. During preparations for the Beijing Women's Conference, for example, many embryonic women's networks gained legitimacy by organizing and summarizing the results of countrywide consultations with women's and other civil society organizations. Many networks then became part of the official negotiations and, in some cases, members of country delegations.

Within the framework of global policy processes stimulated by the UN summits, the Latin American women's rights movement secured significant national policy successes in the 1980s and 1990s. Fourteen Latin American countries ratified the Convention on the Elimination of All Forms of Discrimination Against Women (CEDAW), and twenty-five Latin American and Caribbean countries ratified the 1994 Inter-American Convention on the Prevention, Punishment, and Eradication of Violence Against Women (Belém Convention). Following the Belém Convention, national movements were instrumental in securing the passage of legislation against violence against women in most Latin American countries, although the quality and enforcement of the legislation is uneven.[14] All Latin American countries joined in the consensus for the 1994 ICPD Programme of Action and the 1995 FWCW Plan of Action. Most took a variety of measures to bring their population policies and health systems in line with the recommendations of ICPD and many established women's bureaus or ministries as recommended by FWCW. In addition, several national movements have succeeded in passing new legislation on sexual violence and/or sexual harassment.[15]

The Reproductive and Sexual Rights Advocacy Agenda in Latin America

Post-ICPD, most Latin American states officially accepted their obligation to provide reproductive health services for those segments of the population unable to access services through other means. In general, reproductive health statistics have improved in the region, due in part to increased access to and acceptance of contraceptive services for adult women plus renewed investment in noncontroversial measures to reduce maternal mortality. However, access to these services is in jeopardy. Fertility rates fell markedly in the 1980s and 1990s, and so external donors whose main interest is population control have mostly withdrawn from the region. With regard to sexual health, the HIV/AIDS epidemic is "well established and in danger of spreading both more quickly and more widely in the absence of effective responses."[16] Mediated by processes of health-sector reform and the rise of religious fundamentalism, governments' ability and political will to provide sufficient funding for sexual and reproductive health services are limited.[17]

Since 2000, the major issues remaining on the agenda of the sexual/reproductive rights movement have become more contentious. In 2002, several regional advocates and donors[18] noted the relative lack of progress toward expanding the legal causes for abortions.[19] Beginning in 2001, the reinstatement of the "Global Gag Rule"[20] by the administration of U.S. President George W. Bush has had a chilling effect on public advocacy for liberalizing abortion laws on the part of any organizations receiving U.S. government funds. Progress varies widely from country to country on other issues, such as elimination of discrimination on the basis of HIV status and sexual orientation, and access to a range of sexual and reproductive health products and services: condoms, contraception and sex education for adolescents, emergency contraception, abortions in situations where they are legal, prevention education on HIV/AIDS, and medicines for those living with HIV/AIDS.[21] The Catholic Church and the religious right pose serious political roadblocks to progress on all issues except access to medicines for those living with HIV/AIDS.

Taking the regional view, on the issue of abortion in particular, the widespread perception among advocates is that the women's and reproductive rights movement is losing the communications battle with social forces against reproductive rights.[22] The following interrelated trends help to explain the relative lack of progress:

• the decline in support by donors in the United States and Europe for Latin American NGOs and their networks working on women's issues and reproductive rights;

• the inability of these NGOs to secure alternative sources of support from within their countries, resulting in the weakening and/or disappearance of many NGOs and networks;

• increased activism and communications campaigns opposed to reproductive rights issues, in particular by the Catholic Church and other conservative religious groups and organizations;

• the dearth of proactive strategies for reproductive rights that could take back the initiative from the religious right; and

• failure to expand the constituencies that actively support sexual and reproductive rights.

In the face of decreasing financial support, feminist NGO networks have perceived the need to have proactive public policy strategies, increase their exposure in the communications media, and expand their constituencies. In 2002, several national and regional network initiatives responded to these strategic challenges. Some notable examples are the Campaign for a Convention for Sexual and Reproductive Rights, with sixteen regional networks and national NGOs;[23] the recently formed Latin American Consortium on Emergency Contraception, with more than thirty NGO or agency members in the United States and Latin America; La Alianza—a pro-choice consortium in Mexico, with two international and three national NGOs spearheading an ambitious effort to expand pro-choice constituencies;[24]

and campaigns in several countries—Brazil is the best-known example—to expand the availability of those abortions that already are legal.[25]

Professional Organizations in Social Movements: Advocacy NGOs and Networks in Latin America

On the national level, the structure, financial situation, and constituencies of many Latin American NGOs in the 1990s and early 2000s pose barriers to effective advocacy. In brief, the professional-technical character of the organizations complicates their insertion in a social movement.[26]

The main women's and reproductive rights NGOs are staffed professional feminist groups—some of which specialize in health issues—that depend on foreign funding and state contracts for their work to benefit the most vulnerable sectors of the population, in most cases low-income women. The NGOs shrink and expand to the extent that they are able to secure projects or contracts.

In a context of rapidly declining international cooperation in Colombia and Chile during the 1990s and 2000s, many of the NGOs in this study were in crisis. Chile enjoyed generous "solidarity funding" for a large and diverse NGO sector during the military dictatorship (1973–1990); then external aid to NGOs decreased precipitously during the 1990s, leading to the extinction of many NGOs and to severe financial stress for others. The women's NGOs with more international connections and programs in public policy research fared better than NGOs working at the community level.[27] Although Colombian NGOs also suffered sharp decreases in external aid in the 1990s and early 2000s and found themselves in financially precarious straits, they were never as dependent on international aid[28] as the Chileans, and the concept of voluntary activism (*militancia*) was more firmly entrenched in the culture of women's NGOs.[29]

Unfortunately, for Latin American NGOs that engage in political advocacy on controversial issues such as human rights, land reform, or sexual and reproductive health, national philanthropy cannot easily take the place of lost sources of international support. The philanthropic sector in most Latin American countries is expanding, but only occasionally moves beyond a traditional charitable or, more recently, an antipoverty or community development focus.[30] Women's advocacy NGOs that also provide services, such as counseling for victims of rape or domestic violence or sex education programs for the local schools, have better chances of finding local sources of support. Direct support for social change, whether at the policy or grassroots level, is scarce. According to Cynthia Sanborn, "Few elite or corporate donors support NGOs working in social and economic development, and virtually no national philanthropy goes to those civil society organizations most directly involved in the effort to promote democracy, defend human rights and hold government accountable for its actions."[31] Consequently, except in rare cases, the NGOs' ability to engage in advocacy depends on the willingness of already overburdened staff to engage in nonfunded activities.[32]

Although NGO staff members can use networks to activate their many informal links to other like-minded NGOs and individuals for campaigns on specific issues, these links do not support their NGOs financially, and the other NGOs in the network compete for the same scarce funding sources. This competition can complicate efforts to form solid advocacy networks or coalitions and, indeed, poses an obstacle to fund-raising for coalitions.

Since NGO advocacy staff members are mainly middle-class professionals, some have social and familial connections to political and financial elites. However, they rarely use these connections to benefit their programs. Social movements by definition fall outside the framework of institutional political systems.[33] The movements for women's rights and for sexual and reproductive rights are relatively marginalized from political parties or other centers of power.[34] As such, they rely almost entirely on what political network theorist David Knoke calls "persuasive" power,[35] as opposed to "coercive" or "authoritative" power. The networks' persuasive power relies on their ability to use their arguments to influence the media (another source of persuasive power) and key national and international actors (for example, sympathetic legislators or judiciary) who have authoritative power.

When NGO staff members fail to activate whatever personal networks they may have among elites, they limit their potential for political and financial support. Gerald Marwell, Pamela Oliver, and Ralph Prahl reviewed a number of studies of collective action suggesting that "heterogeneous groups with more centralized networks are better able to mobilize resources from potential participants through ... the number of people an individual could directly organize .... Sheer size of personal networks, not the strength or weakness of ties, dwarfed all other factors' contributions to successful or failed mobilizations."[36]

Analysis of donor and government patterns of support may be another factor in the NGOs' relative marginalization from local elites or centers of power. Due to donor and government priorities, the projects and contracts that fund the NGO members of the networks in this study focus on and benefit low-income women *outside* the NGO staffs' personal networks. Thus, any mobilization of personal networks—which have more political clout because they tend to include middle- and upper-income individuals— assumes a lower priority because it is an unfunded activity. Consequently, most Latin American women's rights and sexual and reproductive rights NGOs have failed to build a substantial constituency of middle- and high-income individuals who could provide both financial and political support. One hypothesis that emerges from this study of NGO networks is that this failure is a key obstacle to successful advocacy for the organizations and their networks, heightening their financial and political vulnerability as they address highly controversial issues.

As noted above, despite their relative marginalization from political elites, NGO networks have gained some access to international, regional, and national policymaking spheres, often linked to UN summit processes. NGO networks seemed a logical choice for inclusion in country delegations, especially when they coordinated national consultations leading to the summits. In other instances when governments decide to involve "civil society" in some policy forum, NGO networks also seem to be a logical choice because their membership includes many organizations. NGO networks can legitimately claim to represent a broader range of voices and experiences than any one organization, and this claim often provides them a seat at the table in national or international policymaking processes.

However, this logic of representing sectors of civil society is quite problematic because NGO networks are not broad membership organizations. Korzeniewicz and Smith say that international labor leaders often refer to NGO activists as NGIs or "non-governmental individuals."[37] In short, a mismatch exists between the professional character of the organizations and their insertion in social movements. The NGO network leaders in this study are aware that they cannot claim to represent "civil society" or even the women's movement:

Representation is a complex and difficult problem, because who do NGOs represent? Only themselves. ... And what about the individuals who participate in networks [that mainly include NGOs]? ... So representation is a new problem, because most of our experiences are with confederations that more clearly represent the voice of large groups of citizens, such as political parties and trade unions[38]

Who decides which member of a network sits at the table, especially when the network encompasses diverse trends and sectors? The processes for such choices are not always transparent. Often, provincial and low-income grassroots (*sector popular*) organizations are excluded from these few instances of NGO networks' access to spheres of influence.

This study revealed other representation problems in venues such as the International AIDS Conferences and regional or global women's conferences. First, often the donors to a conference weigh in on who gets to attend, and so CSOs with few contacts among donors rarely attend. Second, global networks are set up at global meetings, and so the leadership—including the regional or country representatives—consists of those who had the funds and the time to attend. Third, global NGO meetings are usually in English, and so non-English-speakers are underrepresented. In summary, the representation issues for regional and global conferences and networks are also of great concern. Individual NGO leaders and/or their organizations accumulate disproportionate power within their movements on this basis, creating competitive tensions within the movement.

The following section will describe the main advocacy strategies carried out by these Latin American NGO networks during the 1990s and early 2000s, as described by the participants in this study.

Main Advocacy Strategies of the Latin American NGO Networks

Latin American NGO networks have adopted varied advocacy strategies, working with diverse audiences, such as community groups, schools, health services, governmental commissions, the courts, legislatures, and the mass media. A full description of the political strategies employed by these networks and an analysis of their effectiveness would require another paper in itself.[39] In general, the strategies have fallen into one or more of the following categories: (1) direct communications with decision-makers, public educators, and members of the media; (2) public/private partnerships; and (3) constituency-building, including alliances and coalitions with other networks or organizations. The following points will only briefly note significant aspects of the strategies identified in the study.[40]

Participation in the Days of Action Established in the Calendars of the Women's Movement[41]

One hundred percent of the groups interviewed at the provincial, national, and regional levels have adopted this most popular strategy. The networks universally observe three of the days of action: March 8, International Women's Day; May 28, International Day of Action for Women's Health; and November 25, International Day against Violence against Women. Many, but not all, NGO networks in the study also plan events around September 28, the Latin American and Caribbean Day for Decriminalization of Abortion, and World AIDS Day on December 1. For these days of action, the networks' members engage in media events, public meetings, educational events, and fairs, often in multisectoral coalitions with both public and private partners. The days of action have proved to be a useful way to structure educational activities, lobbying, and outreach to the public, using the diverse and complementary resources available to a network to good effect. A few of those interviewed, however, criticized overreliance on the days of action as indicating a lack of long-term strategic planning and clear advocacy objectives.

Monitoring of International Agreements such as the ICPD Programme of Action and the FWCW Platform for Action

This is the second most popular political strategy among the networks, possibly because they participated in the UN summits that produced these agreements. The advocacy groups have been involved in monitoring their governments and demanding accountability for the actions in the agreements. Some networks or NGO members are involved in partnerships with governments to help them translate the agreements into the design of programs on the ground. For example, in Peru, the monitoring of ICPD takes place within the framework of a "Tripartite Commission" that includes NGOs, universities, government officials, and donor agencies; this mechanism gives feminist advocates ample opportunity to engage in dialogue with government officials regarding policy proposals.

However, these are consensus documents and do not create binding obligations for the governments who sign them. They do not have the status of international human rights treaties, which, when ratified, create binding obligations on governments. This study only found three examples of use of international human rights treaty bodies or regional human rights commissions by the networks. This seems to be an important gap in the strategies of these networks.[42]

Training of Health-Sector and Other Professionals

This is the main strategy used by feminist and reproductive health NGOs to assist governments and other programs to translate the principles of ICPD and FWCW into concrete improvements in programs. The expertise of these NGOs is in demand in issues such as gender, sexual and reproductive health and rights, violence against women, quality of care, and adolescent programs. Other categories of professionals trained include judges, lawyers, police, secondary school teachers, and journalists. These NGOs usually employ Freirian[43] participatory training methods, a mode of engagement with the health sector that has proved to be mutually beneficial.[44]

Establishing a Meta-Network

Colombian groups established a "network of networks" in order to coordinate actions among diverse networks that share general goals, such as social justice, human rights, peace, and women's empowerment. This strategy potentially increases the constituency—in this case, the base of support among other activists—for the controversial issues espoused by reproductive rights networks.

Provision of Expertise and Research

In Colombia and Peru, NGO network members testified in several instances before congressional committees; court appearances were less frequent. Some networks carried out public opinion polls, documentation of rights abuses, analyses of legal frameworks, evaluations of quality of care in health services, or epidemiological studies to document the extent of a sexual or reproductive health problem. Such strategies are suitable for the project-based funding generally available from international donors, although the projects often include insufficient time or funds for the ample dissemination that would take full advantage of the investment in research. Networks used the research both for media campaigns and for direct communications with decision-makers.

Legislative Campaigns[45]

The recent examples cited in this study were reactive campaigns, mostly by ad hoc networks, to thwart initiatives by socially conservative sectors to impose more limitations on sexual and reproductive rights. In all countries that drafted a new constitution in the 1990s, for example, conservatives attempted to include a clause protecting the life of the embryo from the time of conception. In Chile, ad hoc networks blocked attempts to increase criminal penalties for abortion. Examples of more proactive campaigns include those of the Inter-American Convention on Sexual and Reproductive Rights, a new NGO network in Chile championing the passage of a Sexual and Reproductive Rights bill in the Congress, and a multisectoral coalition in Colombia backing a bill to decriminalize abortion.[46]

Involvement in Multisectoral Committees

These committees are public/private partnerships in which the full range of organizations active in a given municipality or region pool their resources toward implementing jointly planned strategies, often with an annual work plan. Multisectoral committees convened by the health sector proliferate in Peru,[47] while Colombia's decentralization reform has created municipal, provincial, and national planning commissions. Such committees give evidence of a new, more collaborative relationship between the state and civil society organizations, and they function best when state decision-making is decentralized to the local and regional levels. In the absence of such committees, NGO networks commonly engage in multisectoral meetings and events to publicize issues and campaigns.

Publicity and Legal Campaigns Defending a Victim of Rights Abuse

The Internet has been widely used for this purpose in the past decade, with excellent results among those sectors with access to computers. When cases are particularly compelling, as in the cases of Alba Lucia in Colombia and Paulina in Mexico,[48] this can be an extremely powerful strategy to expand the social base of a network, as long as the network has the ability to manage growth.

Media Outreach

In this region, radio proves to be the media most accessible to the input of NGOs, much more so than television and newspapers. The Cali chapter of the Colombian Women's Network for Sexual and Reproductive Rights (Red Colombiana de Mujeres por los Derechos Sexuales y Reproductivos—CWNSRR) found that its constituency and legitimacy increased noticeably with weekly radio programs aired over the course of two years. In this study, media in provincial cities seemed to be more open to the inclusion of content provided by NGOs than the media in national capitals.

Ad Hoc Coalitions

Broad-based coalitions convoke adherents to a campaign on an ad hoc basis when rapid action is necessary to achieve clearly defined political objectives. One of the main conclusions from this study, to be discussed later in this chapter, is that such ad hoc coalitions can serve the need for rapid political response better than an institutionalized NGO advocacy network and can reach out to a broader network of possible supporters.

Public Pronouncements in Response to Rights Abuses or Critical Political Junctures in Reproductive Rights Advocacy

Many advocates view this strategy as the indispensable criterion for what an advocacy network should do. Both outside observers and network members believe that if a network does not make a timely public statement, it has failed in its central mission. *In fact, this was the most difficult strategy for the NGO networks to carry out.* The following sections on internal governance and managing of growth and diversity will explore the reasons for this difficulty.

BENEFITS OF THE NETWORKS

"Networks entangle us, but they have opened many doors."

With this statement, Beatriz Quintero of the National Women's Network in Colombia succinctly summed up the costs and benefits of NGO networks. In effect, the women's rights and reproductive rights movements in Latin America have made an investment in networking to increase their political impact. This study examines how the networks are "tangled" in their strategic decision-making; however, it is important to put the analysis into perspective. Obviously, those who have elected to stay in the networks have weighed the costs and benefits and found that the latter preponderate. NGOs join forces to achieve increased strength in numbers, to pool resources and share division of labor, and to gain a myriad of tangible and intangible benefits listed below. An examination of the benefits sheds some light on why the current members persist in spite of the problems and why NGO networks continue to proliferate.

In the author's experience, NGOs abandon advocacy networks for three main reasons: (1) internal crises in the NGO, generally when institutional survival was threatened; (2) lack of funding and lack of a paid coordinator, which lower the activity level of the network; and (3) frustration with dysfunctional internal dynamics that lead to lack of political action, lack of internal solidarity among the members, and acute conflicts with no clear resolution. In some cases, internal conflicts have led to the dissolution of a network. The experiences of the networks examined in this study suggest that when networks are functioning well, that is, when leaders continue to organize activities viewed as important, the members remain committed, in spite of lack of funding and the demands that entail burdensome time commitments.

A diverse and shared list of benefits perceived by members of these NGO networks shows how the networks strengthen members as institutions, and, in the long-term, benefit advocacy for recognition of women's rights and sexual and reproductive rights. The report of a Ford Foundation meeting of advocacy groups summed up these benefits quite well:

The participants agreed that networks provide enormous advantages to advocacy work both on the national and regional level. In effect, they increase the impact of the actions of their members. They have an important demonstration effect, that is, they allow members to compare and validate local experiences with regional frameworks. They are useful instruments to exercise political pressure. Networks and coalitions offer greater credibility, sustainability, impact, and access to holistic, comprehensive strategies. The networks maximize the full potential of the available resources, and increase the capacity to carry out public campaigns and apply political pressure.[49]

The chief benefits of networks cited by the networks in this study include the following:

- *Increased visibility and success of political initiatives and campaigns* were signaled in many accounts that related how the complementary efforts of diverse groups within a network came together to increase the political impact of a campaign.

- *Increased legitimacy* results when policymakers and other important social actors perceive NGO members as part of a larger representative group. Funding agencies tend to view network membership as a plus—an indicator that an NGO cooperates with its peers. In Colombia, planning commissions invite NGO networks to participate as representatives of the women's movement. However, this can lead to representation problems when a network has little national reach.

- *Active cooperation with regional, national, and international advocacy campaigns* provides important sources of solidarity and legitimacy for national-level efforts and lessens the isolation experienced by many organizations and activists when working on controversial topics related to gender, sexuality, and reproduction.

- *Access to information and educational materials on topics pertinent to the network is* traditionally provided by most networks, and its importance should not be underestimated. The communications revolution in electronic mail and the Internet has facilitated access enormously, at least among urban NGOs.

- *Interchange with organizations working on similar issues* enriches NGO programs. "Institutions become stale, losing their ability to be surprised. When they enter the Network, they can be surprised by what others are doing, and energized by comparing and sharing.... It is like breathing fresh air. They share solutions to problems, and can see beyond their noses." [50]

- *Connections between provincial NGOs and capital-based NGOs* have several positive effects. Provincial NGOs are strengthened through the network's access to information and resources, and they gain access to national forums to represent their concerns.

- *Access to training* is provided by all of the networks. Training is essential when network members confront a new or difficult issue and when an introduction to the political issues and principles of the network is needed for new members.

- *Access to financial assistance for individual study and for NGO programs and campaigns* can be increased, either through sharing of information on funding opportunities or through channeling funds received by the network to members for projects or campaigns. This increased access is especially significant for the grassroots and/or provincial NGO members.

- *Access to financial assistance for attendance at national, regional, and international conferences* can provide a linkage to regional and international movements for formerly isolated NGOs outside of capital cities, assuring important connections and information that previously were unavailable.

However, network members provided numerous anecdotes of competitive tensions unleashed in the distribution of these benefits, causing disruption in the network. A network's leaders can monopolize any of these benefits, thus exacerbating a climate of competition among members and creating a privileged class within the network. Obstacles exist to equitable distribution of benefits between provincial and grassroots groups on the one hand, and capital-based NGOs on the other (See discussion in the section below: Incorporating Provincial Organizations). Organizing the flow of important information equitably among members takes someone's time, and that time is not always available. A paid network coordinator helps to ensure equity in access to information and other benefits.

Increased access to financial assistance, training, and conferences can cause severe competitive tensions when the process and criteria for choosing the recipients of the benefits are not transparent. Decisions to appoint particular groups or individuals as representatives of the network in important political arenas are fraught with competition because of the increased legitimacy enjoyed by the appointee. While NGOs value their connections with international and regional campaigns, all recognize that these often drain scarce human and financial resources from NGO members and from their work with national constituencies. Finally, the achievements of a network can mask the contributions of each NGO member, making it difficult for an NGO to report successes to its donors; this "dilution" provides incentives for network members to make their participation stand out in ways that exclude other network members.

The following section will analyze the internal governance structures and dilemmas of the networks in this study and discuss how these structures might influence the networks' decision-making abilities.

CHALLENGES IN THE INTERNAL GOVERNANCE OF NGO NETWORKS

As late as 1995, Joe Foweraker remarked, "Enduring coalitions between [professionalized] social movement organizations (SMOs)[51] remain rare" partly due to the presence of "counter-movements and competing SMOs." In Latin America, the NGO advocacy network is a relatively new phenomenon, and scant literature addresses the networks' internal governance at the national level.[52] However, the U.S. literature[53] on interest group and legislative coalitions mentions many of the issues that emerged in the present study, as follows:

1. the challenge of building trust and unified stands among diverse organizations;
2. the need to manage different levels of involvement of organizations in the coalition;
3. the need to build intermediary decision-making structures as the coalition expands and matures; and
4. the trade-off between expansion and diversity on the one hand, and the ability to take united stands on controversial issues, on the other.

The main challenge in the internal governance of advocacy networks relates to the task of stimulating united action among diverse organizations through productive management of conflicts and tensions, which are inevitable in organizational networks or coalitions. The tensions intensify when the coalitions involve any of the following: different socioeconomic classes, majority and minority ethnic groups, very diverse organizations, public and private organizations, or complex and polarized political environments. Each new advocacy network must learn how to manage these tensions productively in order to meet its political goals. Most networks find that in order to manage this diversity and decisions, they need to institutionalize along several dimensions discussed in this section.

Aspects of Institutionalization

Ways of organizing NGO networks vary widely. Yet all networks face certain common issues and decisions as they move from a loose movement structure toward institutionalization or "bureaucratization"[54] to become more efficient and effective. They must decide on the founding mission and principles, legal structure and bylaws, lines of authority and democratic procedures, membership structure, coordination structure, and financial sustainability strategies. The networks in this study varied along all these dimensions. However, three aspects of institutionalization—authority structures with decision-making rules, defined membership structures, and financial sustainability—seem to be key factors in a network's ability to respond adequately to political crises and opportunities, and will be discussed at length.

The evidence in this study suggests that the relationship between the other dimensions of institutionalization and a network's effectiveness in political advocacy is far from straightforward. For example, the National Forum of Women and Population Policy in Mexico, established to monitor the government's compliance with the ICPD Programme of Action, decided not to incorporate legally, with little adverse effect on its ability to act in the policy arena or receive financial support. In Peru, in one case discussed later in this study, an informal ad hoc network with no legal standing has been more agile and timely than institutionalized networks in responding to political controversies over reproductive rights.

Membership

The question of membership is complex in NGO networks and, to some extent, the situations are different for regional and national networks. Four networks in this study consciously limit growth; new NGO members either have to apply or be invited to join.[55] Only two regional networks, which have been in existence since the mid-1980s, have different levels of membership depending on level of participation. The larger national networks lack formal membership procedures, and only one network collects dues from the members. National networks tend to suffer from ambiguity about membership; organizations drop in and out of regular attendance at meetings without explicitly saying that they are withdrawing or officially joining. More experienced networks view attendance at local chapter/provincial meetings as the essential criteria for membership.

Several NGO networks in this study add a further level of confusion about membership by also welcoming the participation of unaffiliated individuals. NGO networks are chronically short of people to do their work, and they benefit greatly by inviting individuals who are committed activists in the rights field and who participate fully in the month-to-month activities of a network or a network chapter. Two major unresolved issues are related to the participation of individuals. First, most networks that take formal votes have not decided on the relative weight of individuals' votes as against NGO representatives' votes. In at least one case, individuals have no voting rights; in other cases, individuals can be chosen as delegates from a provincial chapter to a national assembly. Second, some individuals in the group interviews expressed frustration because plans for network activities and meetings tend not to take into account their needs and constraints. NGO staff can take time during the day for network activities because most NGOs view participation in a network as a legitimate use of staff time. Individuals, on the other hand, may work full time and have to fit their activism into their nonworking hours. They also pay their own expenses related to network participation. These relative disadvantages can lead to demoralization of individual volunteers in a network unless the network recognizes their level of sacrifice and facilitates their participation.

Some network leaders point out that the whole concept of "membership" does not fit well with the character of present-day social movements. In reality, most social movement organizations count mainly on *militantes*—a small number of committed activists who always come to the meetings—and then several levels of supporters:

Although it is true that there are few women in the [National Women's] Network, we understand this as a problem characterizing modern social movements, where there are few militants, but around them there are more women who do not participate all of the time, but who can be counted on [to participate in the Network initiatives].[56]

Two of the regional networks—CLADEM and LACWHN—have institutionalized different levels of membership in order to recognize different levels of commitment to the network's activities, but as of 2000, none of the national networks in this study had done so. Although some national network leaders referred to tensions related to the "free riders" in the network, that is those members not doing their share of the work, the major conflicts did not revolve around this issue, which is so prominent in the early academic literature on collective action.[57]

Institutionalization of criteria and procedures for membership can be an important step forward for an NGO network, facilitating decision-making, transparency in the distribution of benefits, and adjustment of benefits to levels of commitment and participation, while helping to legitimize a network's claims to represent the views of member organizations and individuals.

Authority and Rotation of Leadership

A trade-off occurs between expanding the number of members with decision-making authority and increasing the efficiency of decision-making. Amparo Claro, former coordinator of the LACWHN, expressed this tension succinctly: "To what extent should we democratize, without becoming so democratic that we cannot take action?" All the networks in this study have struggled to decide where to land on the continuum between sharing decision-making as broadly as possible among all the members and restricting decision-making to staff and/or elected representatives. The first tendency is more inclusive and empowering of the membership, but, when taken to the extreme, often results in slow and conflictive decision-making processes and/ or in lack of transparency because the actual authority structures are hidden and unofficial. The second tendency results in more efficient and transparent decision-making, but, when taken to the extreme, can result in entrenched power elites and in the exclusion of significant membership groups from decision-making.

All these networks with their base in the women's movement embraced the first inclusive tendency in their early stages; this seemed to hamper their ability to take political action on risky and controversial issues. Several networks have the annual assembly of members as the maximum decision-making body that makes important policy decisions and exercises financial oversight. However, the latter function suffers under this system. Lacking an external board of directors, these networks (and many NGOs) displace the financial oversight function onto their paid staff and donors, and often the members have no financial committee.[58]

Another disadvantage of the membership assembly as the maximum decision-making body is that its representativity depends on funding for travel and meeting expenses. Some national networks have an easier time securing funding for membership plenary meetings than do the regional networks, both because national meetings cost less and because certain countries, such as Peru, still enjoy more sources of international support than do others, such as Colombia, Argentina, and Chile. In smaller networks, such as the post-Beijing groups, whose core members are all from the national capital, the membership could meet as often as every two weeks. Larger national networks that actively involve provincial members may meet only once a year, or simply when funding permits; in these cases, having the membership as the decision-making body is unwieldy, and most of these networks eventually elect a steering or executive committee. However, when the steering committee represents groups from different provinces, financing and managing the logistics of coordination is a challenge as well.

Several networks evidenced confusion about the degree of authority invested in the representative to the network by each NGO. Serious obstacles to effective decision-making result when representatives who attend the meetings cannot make decisions on behalf of their organizations. Smaller networks, such as Peru's post-Beijing network, solve this problem by demanding that the director of each NGO attend the meetings, or if not the director, then someone to whom she has delegated decision-making power.

The regional networks, on the other hand, have been in existence longer and have received donations to help organize UN summit-related advocacy; they thus tend to be more institutionalized. They have an official advisory board or executive committee, legal status as nonprofit institutions, and bylaws governing rotation of coordinators and the board or steering committee. The difficulty and expense of organizing regional meetings means that these networks rarely have membership meetings, which are costly, and so a steering committee and staff make most decisions. The two that have regular regional meetings are those that limit their membership—CLADEM, meeting every three years, and Catholics for the Right to Decide, every year. For a regional organization, having the advisory board or executive committee meet regularly is a large expense in itself.[59]

One important way to organize decision-making in a network is to adopt bylaws with procedures for rotation of board members and coordinators, so that no one person or organization "owns" the network. The networks in this study covered the entire range of possibilities. Only one network has had the same coordinator and coordinating NGO practically since its inception;[60] others have regularly rotated coordinators. When CLADEM rotated coordinators, this meant that the coordinator was based in Argentina while the central office of the organization remained in Peru. Such arrangements have become workable only recently, with the advent of electronic communications.

In summary, any network that cannot have regular membership meetings must reduce the size of the decision-making group. In the absence of institutionalized procedures, in several cases in this study, authority has devolved informally to self-appointed leaders or founders, usually from the capital city or the regional office.

Moving from Consensus to Decision Rules

On one end of the spectrum, the majority of the national networks interviewed reported that they make their decisions by consensus. Many networks either do not question this rule or are only beginning to contemplate change. Several clarified that while consensus is the preferred modus operandi, the majority prevails when the majority view is strong with few dissenters. Reflecting on the early stages in a network's trajectory, several experienced network activists commented that they constructed decision-making rules after the first instances of conflict signaled the need to move beyond consensus rules. Teresa Valdés described the problems in the early stages of the Post–Beijing Initiative Group in Chile: "We are very different organizations, so that making a collective declaration was very difficult. We didn't do anything in which we had not reached agreement, we did everything by consensus."

At the other end of the spectrum, CLADEM adheres to parliamentary procedures; possibly, its members' training as lawyers makes them more comfortable with this mode of decision-making than most feminist organizations.

In voting, we use the system of absolute majority, 50 percent, plus one. We believe that seeking consensus is not only undemocratic, but [also] authoritarian since with a consensus system a single person [or institution] can block or hinder the decisions of the immense majority of members.[61]

This observation is verified by the experience of one Peruvian network. Facing a strong difference of opinion about whether or not to invite a prominent minister to an event, only one organization disagreed with the invitation, and the minister was not invited.

One activist explained her theory of the primacy of the consensus rule: "Networks arose 30 years ago with the feminist movement as collectives of individuals, but now the networks are made up of NGOs. The problem is that the networks haven't adapted to their new composition."[62] Another common explanation is that female socialization causes women to place high value on cooperative interpersonal links and relationships, and so networks dominated by women will give high priority to the quality of relationships[63] within the group and the cohesiveness of the group, in some cases sacrificing the political principle at stake in any given disagreement. While some cases support the latter theory, others do not. In many cases, dissenting members left the network rather than sacrifice their political principles, while others stayed within, but engaged in ongoing conflicts.

Several network members pointed out that operating by consensus is an important obstacle to producing public statements from the network. "Organizations sign [letters to the authorities] as organizations, and when there are disagreements, sometimes we haven't known how to handle them. For a regional network, having only some members of the network sign is difficult."[64]

When unexpected events demand a political and public response, an NGO network can prove to be a cumbersome instrument at best. Typically, the most public ways that networks engage in policy debates are through paid declarations in the written press, letters to public officials, or press releases and conferences on breaking issues. Increasingly, network representatives have gained more exposure in radio and television programs. As the quotes above point out, NGO networks often find it logistically and politically difficult to produce public declarations. Either too many parties are involved in the editing, or they cannot reach agreement on some key aspect of the declaration or letter.

Some institutions need to study [public declarations] more before acting. This makes the collective process very slow, and just when one believes that everything is set, someone decides that the tone of the communication needs to be adjusted.[65]

In one instance in Colombia, the NGO in charge of communications within the network unilaterally eliminated all mention of abortion from a communiqué on safe motherhood. This so angered other network members that some key organizations quit, almost causing the dissolution of the network. This case illustrates the role of the degree of controversy surrounding the issue at hand—a key contributor to the difficulty in reaching agreement.

"With some obvious issues, there are no problems in reaching consensus."[66] For issues such as violence against women, networks commonly authorize the coordinator or a representative to draft and sign public communications in the name of the network members. In general, however, public communications are difficult to produce in these NGO networks when the issue involves abortion or an initiative that might incur political risks for network members by bringing them into confrontation with government entities. This study analyzes the relationship between decision-making and political costs in detail in the section below on financial stresses and political risks.

Although rules for decisions are necessary, they are not sufficient. Constructing agreement in any coalition or network is an interpersonal process, and the application of the decision-making rules is the final moment in the process. NGO networks need to hold complex, multifaceted conversations to address political differences, to agree on common principles and goals, to construct sound political strategies, and to build trust among the members so that the network can better weather the tensions that inevitably arise in organizational networks. The highly controversial nature of certain issues in sexual and reproductive rights increases the tensions in discussions on political strategy. Such discussions best take place face to face.

Now [after the last National Assembly] the relationships between us have changed and we are friends. No one wants to miss the Assembly. Face-to-face meetings are important. The last assembly helped us to grow, to be more committed; it is a vital space for interchange.[67]

The literature on political coalitions[68] and many network members point out that there is no substitute for face-to-face meetings. Regular membership meetings serve the important function of building interpersonal trust. Such exchanges can begin or continue via e-mail, but face-to-face conversations produce resolutions and decisions more efficiently when dealing with complex issues and diverse opinions.

Global networks and the Latin American regional networks have taken advantage of the revolution in electronic communications to foster dialogue among members, but with important limitations. Groups from small cities and grassroots networks or organizations are underrepresented because they have less access to computers and the Internet. In addition, the nature of the medium does not allow for efficient interchanges on complex issues and decisions.

The experiences of the Latin American and Caribbean Feminist Network against Domestic and Sexual Violence illustrate the need for face-to-face meetings. Since the late 1990s, the network has been unable to secure funds to hold its regional meeting, although funds have been available for time-limited activities such as the "16 days of activism against gender violence."[69]

[I]f [this network] has no money, it loses momentum without being able to have conversations about structure, and about political action.... UNIFEM has supported us for electronic interchange about strategies, but one cannot resolve some things through e-mail. We take advantage of other [regional or global] meetings to have a quick network meeting, but not everyone who should be there can come. [Under these conditions] it is hard to construct network relationships that are stable and based on concrete initiatives.[70]

The next section will continue to explore the complexities of NGO network decision-making, with a focus on how expansion and diversity— both of which are viewed as intermediate indicators of success for advocacy networks—create challenges for the functioning of the networks.

MANAGING GROWTH AND DIVERSITY

While both donors and advocates view growth and diversity as important objectives, success in achieving these objectives can "entangle" the network unless the accompanying pitfalls are anticipated in planning. The issues of managing growth and diversity are inextricably entwined. When women's rights and reproductive rights networks aim to expand their political influence, many strategies to achieve this goal necessitate expansion beyond their limited constituencies to construct a larger and more diverse NGO network and set of allies.

As most social movements aim to increase their influence, the finding that almost none of the Latin American NGO advocacy networks in this study plan explicitly for expansion in membership and/or social base[71] seems counterintuitive. Two major factors emerged from this study to explain this finding: (1) the inherent challenge in managing growth and (2) the trade-off between broad-based diversity in the membership, on the one hand, and ability to reach agreement efficiently on advocacy strategies, on the other. Greater diversity can erode hard-won consensus on advocacy goals and strategies, especially when the network's issues are socially and politically controversial. This section will explore these two factors but concentrate on the challenges of managing diversity.

Managing Growth

Growth management is a challenge for any organization or business, as evidenced by the vast literature on the topic and the proliferation of consulting companies offering advice on growth strategies to businesses. Network leaders are aware of these challenges. In many cases, NGO members and network staff members already feel so overloaded with their current projects and activities that expending the additional effort required for expansion is unthinkable to them.[72] If growth were to happen, the leaders know that it could overtax their resources. Growth entails increased demands on the NGO's or network's human and financial resources, which usually are fully committed to ongoing projects with restricted (and often insufficient) budgets. Thus, the lack of planning for expansion relates directly to the precarious financial situation of most Latin American NGOs involved in advocacy for women's rights and sexual and reproductive rights, which was mentioned above. This situation is a catch-22, self-defeating cycle in which it is difficult to expand without more funding, and yet it can be equally difficult to attract new sources of support without evidence of "success," such as expansion of the membership or of the social and political base.

Many advocacy NGOs, then, view networks as a manageable way to expand their social base, level of activity, and achievements. The network functions as a political advocacy coalition in which the NGOs pool resources and work toward a common cause, and each can increase its legitimacy by taking some credit with its donors for the network's achievements. However, when the human and financial resources of a network's member NGOs are stretched too thin, the network encounters the same catch-22 cycle of limits to growth as its members. In the absence of a plan for growth, growth "happens" to the network when a particular initiative incites enthusiasm among a wider audience, bringing varying degrees of chaos and overload if the resources are not available to handle expanded demands.

The case of the Alba Lucia Campaign in Colombia (see box 2. 1) illustrates why NGO networks in Latin America often are unable to take advantage of opportunities for growth. This experience illustrates a successful strategy for growth in the social base of the reproductive rights movement and highlights the importance of planning for growth so that the resources needed to manage expansion are in place.

The present study identified several successful examples of a planned growth process in an NGO network, most often linked to the funding opportunities provided by the UN summits. The pre-summit national projects supported both increased public education and consultation with civil society organizations at the provincial level and increased coordination between the network's central headquarters and new provincial chapters or contacts.

However, without donor commitment to ongoing support of the expanded network, any expansion in membership and social base deteriorates over time. The National Women's Network in Colombia and the post-Beijing Initiative Group in Chile, at certain points in the late 1990s, experienced unraveling of their networks when project funding ended.

We are now without any funding at all . . . and it has affected us terribly. . . . In the [provincial] focal points, only the most autonomous are still functioning, while the others have ceased.[73]

Box 2.1
The Alba Lucia Campaign in Columbia

A campaign of the Colombian Women's Network for Sexual and Reproductive Rights (CWNSRR), led by the Medellín chapter from 1997 to 2002 illustrates the challenges posed by unplanned growth resulting from successful advocacy campaigns. In the Alba Lucia Campaign, CWNSRR mobilized both legal and popular support to defend an uneducated, adolescent *campesina* woman who had been gang-raped and became pregnant. She gave birth hidden in her family's latrine, then went into shock, and the baby died. After suffering prejudicial treatment by hospital personnel and police, she was accused of infanticide and condemned to forty-two years in prison.

At first, the Medellín chapter identified a feminist lawyer to defend Alba Lucia pro bono; CWNSRR then undertook a public education campaign of unprecedented dimensions for this network, with a snowball effect that mobilized nationwide audiences rarely involved in reproductive rights campaigns. For example, networks of schoolteachers became involved, with entire classrooms from rural and urban areas of Colombia composing letters to Alba Lucia in prison. The public discussions resulting from this campaign were rich, exposing issues related to adolescents' sexuality, sexual coercion, links between education and reproductive health, voluntary motherhood, and the legal status of abortion. The demand for speakers, the supply of potential volunteers, and the base of potential contributors grew so exponentially that the Medellín network members and their administrative systems were overwhelmed. All but one of the members (the national coordinator of the network) had other jobs and worked on a volunteer basis. The chapter was unable to take full advantage of this unforeseen opportunity for explosive growth in membership and social base.

However, the six-year campaign itself was successful in its main objective. In 2000, CWNSRR entered into partnership with the human rights organization Center for Justice and International Law (CEJIL) to file a complaint against the Colombian government with the Inter-American Human Rights Commission of the Organization of American States (OAS). CWNSRR also pursued its complaint through the Colombian judicial system to the Supreme Court. In March 2002, the Court voided the original sentence and ordered Alba Lucia's release from prison after six years of incarceration.

In some cases, these NGO advocacy networks consider that expansion would hamper their efficiency in decision-making, and they have made a conscious decision not to expand, or to do so very slowly and deliberately. Making a political coalition more broad based may entail either suppressing the more controversial aspects of members' political agendas[74] or broadening the focus to include the diversity of members' agendas.[75] Expanding membership is more problematic than expanding the social base because sudden increases in numbers or diversity of voting network members may revive internal debates that current members consider settled. For the same reasons, the entrance of new members creates an ongoing need for training, which takes time and resources:

When too many new people come to the annual assembly, we have to spend so much time repeating former discussions, giving them information, and persuading them to accept former group decisions, that we cannot move ahead. The challenge is how to expand our social base, train and inform new members, without spending all of our [available] time on this.[76]

It takes time and effort to build a well-functioning leadership team in such a complex undertaking as an advocacy network. These networks, such as the two post-Beijing networks in this study, with a limited membership and a core executive committee in only one city, are painfully conscious of how long it took them to come to agreement on strategies and to learn to work together. They consider the inclusion of any new organizations carefully. After FWCW in Beijing, the Chilean network issued invitations and accepted applications from three NGO members whose focus added important expertise and social bases to the network: two because they work closely with grassroots, low-income groups and one because of its work with youth organizations.

Undoubtedly, the team-building challenge in managing expansion in membership and/or leadership teams is one factor in the "graying of the women's movement," a phenomenon noted by observers in both the United States and Latin America. (The other main factor, of course, is financial/professional self-interest.) Some new Latin American coalitions have NGO leaders who recognize that they are the usual suspects (*las de siempre*), but their shared history of resolving tensions and ideological differences gives them a level of trust that facilitates coalition formation and efficient decision-making processes.[77] This plus, however, must be weighed against the potential minus: the entrenchment of leaders within a movement that fails to renew its strategies and leadership, and to reach out to new sectors of the population and to the next generation.

Managing Diversity

Some of the literature on political coalitions[78] emphasizes multisectorality and diversity as the reasons for the coalitions' "complex, fractious, and fragile" nature.[79] Watts points out that "shared core coalitions" are difficult to generate because "each of the participating sectors of the coalition must relinquish key aspects of [its] own specific agendas in pursuit of a universally shared agenda."[80] As Fred Rose points out:

Building trust and relationships and agreeing to disagree are the ingredients that combine to make diverse coalitions possible. But these are evolving processes-most severely tested at first but requiring wise and conscious development over time if the coalition is to deepen and strengthen.[81]

The present study documented many types of diversity within NGO networks, all of them potential sources of creativity and increased representation on the one hand, and tensions/conflicts on the other. Some networks are multisectoral, including both civil society organizations (CSOs) and representatives from governmental entities. Networks might include CSOs with very distinct focuses and constituencies, including the more professionalized policy/advocacy NGOs, community development NGOs, research centers, university programs, religious groups, and grassroots organizations. Many of the NGO networks in this study include both organizations and individuals. Organizations from different provinces in national networks, and from different countries in regional networks, provide multiple levels of diversity.

However, even networks that are homogeneous on these counts, for example those that include only women's NGOs from one national capital, still struggle to address diverse political ideologies and styles, different levels of political or technical sophistication, and unequal access to financial and human resources among members. In these rights advocacy networks, important sources of diversity include the degree to which the focus of the network coincides with the focus of member NGOs. In particular, financial inequalities and differences in focus on issues lead to differing levels of commitment to the network, creating internal tensions.

Incorporating Grassroots/low-income[82] Organizations

In these rights-focused NGO networks, mainly led by professional staff, a common goal for expansion and diversification of the social base is to include more community-based organizations and networks representing low-income women. Although both the Open Forum for Reproductive and Sexual Health and Rights in Chile and the Colombian CWNSRR have included grassroots women's organizations as full members of their networks, this is the exception rather than the rule. In general, low-income women's organizations do not share the full feminist agenda, especially in sexual and reproductive rights.[83] Their inclusion, therefore, can lead to problems. For example, in 1999, the coordinator of the Bogotá chapter of the CWNSRR represented a grassroots women's network. She personally shared the network's agenda, but she did not have the authority to speak in the name of her organization on controversial issues such as abortion. In Chile, the Open Forum has responded to the challenges of class diversity by investing heavily in training opportunities for provincial members, including several from grassroots organizations. They report that such training allows the intensive give-and-take that is needed to address the strong emotions aroused by sexual and reproductive health and rights issues.

A study of sexual and reproductive rights networks in the United States showed that they are more focused on abortion rights than their Latin

American counterparts, and they have experienced similar issues when attempting to incorporate more low-income women and women from ethnic minorities:

The legal maintenance of abortion rights is generally not a top priority for women with pressing economic needs. Instead, questions of access to health care, including but by no means limited to abortion services, are much more important.... Consequently, it is not surprising that coalitions that have become centrally involved in welfare reform issues... have had much greater success in involving low-income women than those that have focused more narrowly.... Even this, however, is not a panacea.... [T]here are still substantial barriers to including low-income women in coalition work. In particular, the problems of obtaining transportation to meetings and arranging childcare for their duration loom much larger than for middle-class women.... In all three cases [of ethnic minority networks' working on reproductive health], the real and perceived tendency of white-dominated organizations to prioritize abortion rights over all other women's health issues was cited as a fundamental barrier to interracial and interethnic cooperation.[84]

Latin American sexual and reproductive rights and women's rights advocacy networks face similar challenges when incorporating grassroots women's organizations as full partners; their priorities may be different. In some cases, the priorities of the network have expanded as a result. For example, in the National Forum of Women and Population Policy in Mexico, the regional chapter representing Chiapas—a province characterized by a high level of extreme poverty—successfully advocated within the network to give higher priority to demands related to economic justice in the network's monitoring of the implementation of the ICPD Programme of Action.

Divisions of socioeconomic class and ethnicity are a challenge to any NGO network seeking to expand its representation of marginalized sectors of women. Increasing the class and ethnic diversity in membership and in leadership teams requires more dialogue to find common ground and language, more accommodation to differing priorities, and more investment in training, infrastructure, and travel for groups with fewer resources and less technical expertise so that they can participate fully in meetings and in communications between meetings.

These requirements for expanding the scope and representation of a network beyond the NGO staff of professional women also are evident in the findings described below concerning the inclusion of women's organizations from the provinces in national networks.

Incorporating Provincial Organizations

A clear benefit of national networks is that they have the potential to break down centralism and overrepresentation of groups in the capital, which historically have plagued Latin American societies.[85] National networks can give voice to the diversity of needs and interests of the many socioeconomic and cultural groupings within a country. The national networks in this study are divided between those that include provincial representation in decision-making and those whose core NGOs in the capital make the major decisions.[86]

Some significant obstacles to full provincial representation in national networks are linked to the concentration of power and resources in capital cities of most countries and to the ensuing historic tensions between capital and provinces. Ensconced in international and national economic and political structures that privilege a capital city, NGOs in capitals tend to concentrate power and resources to the disadvantage of the provinces, albeit unintentionally. Often, more technically and politically sophisticated organizations in the capital have more access to participation in national policy debates. Through their greater access to international donors, they have more financial resources and access to information. They are more connected with international movements and networks. Coalition theory suggests that such imbalances make most coalitions inherently unstable. "Groups seldom bring equal amounts of political clout or resources to the coalition-building process.... There are few opportunities to equalize the weight of coalition members, thus creating the conditions for instability."[87]

Power and resource imbalances did indeed create tensions in relationships between the capital-based and provincial NGOs that participated in this study. Tensions involved issues of provincial autonomy, representation and funding, and the special disadvantages of rural women's groups.

With the explicit goal of sharing power, the national networks in the study have evolved informal and formal principles of autonomy for provincial chapters. Lucrecia Mesa, former coordinator of the Colombian CWNSRR network, commented: "We have to be pluralist...at the same time as we have a relationship rooted in basic agreements." Within the general initiatives and focuses decided by the network assembly (or by lead NGOs in the case of post–Beijing networks), the provincial groups shape their own campaigns and activities. Although the central coordinating office may produce campaign materials for all chapters, many chapters also produce their own materials adapted to the local context.

This autonomy is especially important in countries with great cultural diversity, as is found in Peru. Another compelling argument for this autonomy is that public opinion about social issues in provincial cities often tends to be more conservative than in the great urban centers, and so the provincial chapters need to have the liberty to decide on appropriate strategies and messages suited to their sociopolitical context. The Open Forum in Chile has a network-wide agreement to promote the principle of "voluntary motherhood"[88] as part of its overall advocacy for reproductive rights and decriminalization of abortion. The metropolitan Santiago chapter appears with banners and flyers one Friday every month in the Plaza de Armas (the city's central plaza) to talk to passersby about legalizing abortion. After a conflictive period in the early stages of the network, the Open Forum coordinators now accept that not all provincial chapters feel prepared, or believe that it is appropriate, to adopt such a public strategy. One of the Open Forum's coordinators elaborated on this point:

Evidently, we cannot impose the pace of change, because there are many ways to conduct advocacy. We are clear that we share the same objectives. We have improved by defining a much more respectful way of working together. For example, if the women from [x province] say to me, "We will not conduct outreach to the mass media on the issue of abortion because it could mean that instead of making progress, we lose ground," then I am capable of respecting the pace of their process, and I do not demand that they engage in this specific activity because they are part of the Forum.

This example from the Open Forum points out a potential problem with the principle of autonomy of chapters within a network. When a chapter consistently refuses to address publicly one of the core goals of a reproductive rights network, in this case, legalization of abortion, at some point is the chapter no longer a member of the network? The regional Catholics for the Right to Decide in Latin America network requires that all members adhere to its statement of principles, which includes support for the legalization of abortion. When one member subsequently failed to adhere to these principles, the result after intense dialogue was that this member left the network. The same tension arose with regard to one of the chapters of the Colombian CWNSRR. The Open Forum's policy of providing intensive training and dialogue on this issue for provincial members is a strategy to bring new members along steadily until they are comfortable with working publicly on the issue. The strategy has worked in some cases.

Another major issue, in addition to autonomy, for provincial chapters in NGO networks relates to funding and representation. The experience of the national networks in this study clearly shows that a network is national in name only when funding is not specifically available for travel to and from provinces, payment of coordinators of provincial networks, communications throughout the national territory, computer access for provincial groups, and activities in the provinces.

For example, the Colombian National Women's Network had excellent provincial representation at its founding meeting. During a period (1998) when the network lost all financial support, its decision-making group was in effect reduced to a core volunteer group of seven women in Bogotá having e-mail contacts with point people (*puntos de enlace*) in certain provincial cities. Although these seven core people still had a broad network of contacts and supporters on whom they could draw for political initiatives, the decision-making group did not represent the true diversity within the network.

Furthermore, the network still enjoyed the legitimacy conferred by supposedly representing the opinions of a national network of NGOs and individuals and was invited to policy debates on that basis. Fortunately, after receiving some minimal support for a national meeting in 1999 and additional funds in 2000, the network recovered and expanded its national representation.[89]

Because of funding constraints, the post–Beijing groups in this study do not include provincial groups in their steering committees and do not pretend to represent groups throughout the country. Members from the provinces could never make a meeting every two to four weeks in the capital. When project funding allows, the core group consults "focal points" in the provinces, and the provincial groups participate in national initiatives. Provincial groups usually come to national meetings only during the planning stage of projects and at closure.

A third major issue, along with provincial autonomy and funding/representation, is the relative lack of access of provincial and rural women to advances in electronic communication, which hold great promise to reduce communication costs for far-flung groups within a country. Quintero again referred to the period when the National Women's Network had no funds: "If we had electronic mail, it would be much better, but many women don't have e-mail. The lack of funds makes communication impossible, which is the heart of a network. This is a serious problem." Isabel Duque, of ISIS, the Initiative Group in Chile, and the Latin American and Caribbean Feminist Network against Domestic and Sexual Violence, provided an update in 2002:

Even though use of electronic mail has increased greatly in our region, the grassroots organizations are still at a disadvantage as compared to the intermediary organizations [NGOs] that work with them. The "telecenters" created in some rural zones have helped to increase access, but women do not necessarily have access to these. The problems for those far from the most important urban centers continue to exist in spite of the recent advances (personal communication with the author).

As Duque pointed out, women in provincial capitals are more marginalized than their capital-based peers; within provinces, however, groups outside the provincial capital suffer even greater marginalization. Rural women simply do not participate in most of these NGO networks. In small cities and rural areas, communications difficulties are much more severe, transport may be expensive or inaccessible, and many groups or individuals have no telephone or fax, much less access to e-mail. Again, the overcoming of these barriers is linked to access to funds:

We are supposedly the network from the fifth region, but actually, we are the network of the province of Valparaiso. We have to make special efforts so that the women from the city of G_____ come, while the women from the city of V_____ have stopped coming and we have to find out why.... For special events like the women's schools [special training events], women from the interior of the region have come, but there is no possibility of forming a network with them. We would need a lot more funds [for transport, etc.].[90]

Other barriers to rural women's participation relate to class and culture:

Women from rural areas feel neither represented nor understood by those in urban areas. Urban organizations are present in the networks, but there are no *campesina* [peasant] women, because they don't feel understood, and because of problems like floods, dangers due to the conflicts, etc., which make access impossible for them.[91]

While advances in communications and computer technology carry the potential of enabling greater connections between urban and rural groups and among groups that are geographically separated, this potential will remain unrealized until both provincial and rural citizens have access to this technology. For now, only the relatively privileged urban organizations enjoy the benefits of connectivity with each other and with global networks at low cost, thus increasing the already considerable social and political distance between them and their rural counterparts. Even given access, other barriers impede this form of network communication. For example, many rural grassroots women have lower literacy levels, with less ability to express themselves in writing or use a keyboard. In addition, the telecenters in rural towns charge for Internet time, creating a financial barrier.

Growth and Diversity: Summary

NGO advocacy networks need to plan for growth in membership, both to expand the sectors working toward their goals and to keep the networks vital. However, balancing the trade-offs of diversity and growth versus focused and efficient action on controversial issues, some NGO networks may decide to remain small advocacy working groups that limit growth in membership and instead focus on expanding their social base and network alliances. The larger national networks that aim to represent many sectors of civil society seek to expand membership, and therefore must orient new members to the basic principles and agreements of the network to avoid needless revisiting of old arguments. However, as membership expands and becomes more diverse, a network will necessarily revisit some previous agreements in order to accommodate the agendas of new sectors, but without sacrificing the basic founding principles.

This discussion has revealed how growth and diversity make decision-making more complex, which in turn makes face-to-face meetings more necessary. Cultural differences among provinces, differences in the agendas of middle-class professionals and low-income women, and the historic mistrust between provinces and capitals make it difficult to create trust and basic agreements without such meetings. When decisions are made at meetings of national networks, grassroots and provincial members cannot be full decision-making partners without some funding for their travel and expenses.

Getting those members to annual network assemblies cannot in itself solve the problem. Network steering committees or coordinators must make crucial decisions between annual meetings, and most networks do not have sufficient funding to include grassroots, provincial, and rural women meaningfully in those committees. Increased access to electronic mail has not yet solved the problem of the relative marginalization of low-income and provincial women. Furthermore, even if the Internet and e-mail were completely available, virtual communication does not work well when complex discussions of political strategy heat up. The conversations taking place through electronic communication are too disjointed, the tone of the written word is too easy to misinterpret, and many women with low literacy levels face too many barriers to participate through these means.

In summary, both growth and diversity in the membership of a network have important consequences both for the network's political agenda and for its ability to reach agreement on strategies. Homogeneous groups and established leadership teams that have learned how to work together over time find it easier to arrive at a consensus on the main goals and focus of a network and on specific responses to political threats and opportunities. The networks need to weigh the benefits against the potential costs of such homogeneity: entrenched leadership, stagnant strategies, and failure to represent well the self-defined needs of diverse sectors of women. To expand and increase diversity, a network must invest in opportunities for dialogue, training, and measures that guarantee access to decision-making spaces.

The next section will analyze how financial stresses create tensions between the interests of NGO members and their NGO networks, and how the political risks associated with controversial issues and/or confrontational strategies further complicate the functioning and strategic decision-making of the networks

FINANCIAL STRESSES AND POLITICAL RISKS

Both the financial sustainability and the political effectiveness of NGO advocacy networks relate closely to the financial health of their members. This study revealed the interplay between the financial stresses facing NGOs in Latin American countries and the ability of networks to be effective protagonists in policy debates. Lack of funds translates into lack of time for networks, and financial vulnerability creates caution. The marked increase in partnerships between the state and the NGO sector has been a source of survival and renewed influence for struggling NGOs, as well as a point of tension within the women's movement in Latin America. Such relationships obstruct the ability of NGOs to act as independent critical voices when the state abuses its power or fails to fulfill its obligations.

Financial Stresses and Conflicts between NGO and Network Interests

One common category of network—for example, a professional association—exists solely for the exchange of information among and professional support for its members, who include both organizations and individuals. This type of network minimizes the possibility of conflict between the interests of the network and its members; by virtue of its mission, the network responds to members' needs.

In contrast, the advocacy networks' *raison d'être* is to achieve long-term political goals shared by members, and only secondarily to benefit the member organizations. Indeed, the political function of NGO advocacy networks entails increased demands on their members and often considerable sacrifices. However, one should not create too sharp a dichotomy between the capacity-building function of professional networks and the political function of advocacy networks. Most advocacy networks also engage in capacity building for their members, who value this function highly. In the long-term, capacity building strengthens advocacy.

In advocacy networks, each member must contribute resources to achieve the shared goals, and when resources for NGOs are scarce, the network suffers disproportionately because advocacy is very time consuming. It demands planning time, difficult political decisions on strategy, and joint activities. When NGO member groups are struggling financially, they are understaffed; they also contribute fewer human and financial resources to network meetings and activities and give lower priority to fund-raising for their network. The decreased commitment by financially pressed members sets into motion a vicious cycle of internal conflicts, declining effectiveness, and loss of sustainability of the network. Internal conflicts exacerbate the already declining participation, leading to diminished public presence. The decrease in public initiatives damages a network's public image, causing it to lose its attractiveness to potential supporters and its legitimacy as a political actor. Due to the sharp decline in external funding for the NGO sector mentioned earlier, especially in Colombia and Chile, this study found several reports of this vicious cycle, which unleashed competition for scarce resources between NGO networks and their members.

NGOs and their advocacy networks are affected not only by declining support, but also by restrictions on the support they receive. When NGOs receive only restricted support for time-bound projects, and not general support, they often must sacrifice long-term projects and goals related to advocacy. A coordinator of the Open Forum in Chile spoke on this point:

The Forum does not have the institutional reserves to allow us freedom of movement as an association. . . . All of the Forum's projects are tied to carrying out specific activities, and the national coordinators' time is consumed with the projects. One of our goals is to find some subsidy so that they could . . . carry out more political outreach and lobbying.

In general, those interviewed agreed that networks have more fund-raising difficulties than their members. NGOs do not want to have a network's fund-raising lessen their chances for support from the limited universe of agencies that give support to women's rights or sexual and reproductive health organizations in Latin America. As was stated in the ISIS group interview, "Without a paid coordinator, there is no one to raise funds for a network. Members' first loyalty is to their NGO. For this reason, it is fundamental that the NGO incorporate network goals and responsibilities as part of its central strategy."

As these leaders noted, an important factor in reducing the competition for fund-raising seems to be the level of correspondence between an NGO's central mission and that of the network. NGOs whose core activities involve activism in the network were more likely to continue to contribute their time and resources even when struggling financially. When the network's focus is not a major component of a NGO member's program, the NGO is more likely to drop out of the network altogether or sharply reduce its commitment. Members of Chile's post-Beijing Initiative Group incorporate their network-related expenses (staff time and direct expenses) into their core funding proposals to donors and recommend this as a strategy to reduce financial conflicts of interest between NGO members and their networks.

This study identified another area of conflicts of interest related to fund-raising. An Open Forum comment about "dilution" of the NGO in a network echoes comments from other networks:

During this period [when funding for Chilean NGOs was drastically reduced], many NGOs were living through dramatic situations, and this change meant that they turned inward. . . . Because in a network your contributions become diluted, and also because of funding . . . these NGOs are not as interested in participating in the network as they used to be because they are totally focused on their survival as institutions.

Part of the "capital" of an NGO is its record of achievements, which is essential for publicity and fund-raising pitches. Even when an NGO has devoted considerable organizational resources to an achievement by a network of organizations, it cannot claim individual credit for it. Some problems that plagued the Community Network to Prevent HIV/AIDS in Chile in the mid-1990s may have been related to the desperate struggle for survival of some member NGOs that organized a major public meeting on their own without including the whole network. This exclusion set off severe internal tensions, with two major founding members leaving the network. These members felt that the others had violated the spirit in which they formed the network by excluding some member organizations in order to better their own position with potential sources of support.[92]

Managing Financial and Political Risks

Women's rights and sexual and reproductive rights NGO networks suffer tensions related to the relationship between civil society organizations and the state. Many of these tensions arise from the adverse political and financial consequences associated with confrontational strategies and advocacy on controversial issues. Given that espousal of controversial reproductive rights initiatives can incur political costs that affect the financial health of NGO members of a network, many NGO advocacy networks have great difficulty in reaching agreement on appropriate political strategies.

Strategic disagreements in these NGO advocacy networks center on a classic social movement tension between "insiders" and "outsiders"; that is, those in favor of negotiating from within mainstream and/or governmental institutions through established procedures versus those favoring "more contestatory strategies."[93] The networks in this study include both types of groups and individuals. This section will examine two key factors in this insider-outsider tension: the NGO members' relationship with the government and the extent to which they focus on the most controversial issues in women's rights and sexual and reproductive rights.

Relationships with Governments

The feminist movement in Latin America suffered severe controversies during the 1990s over the role of the newly professionalized NGOs in the movement and their relationships with governments. The tension built up during regional and national lobbying efforts surrounding the three major United Nations conferences in Vienna, Cairo, and Beijing, where negotiated agreements inevitably led to compromises on some important feminist goals and gave international prominence to certain English-speaking feminist activists. After Beijing, the tension exploded with venom in the Latin American Feminist Meeting in Cartagena in 1996,[94] where "autonomous" feminists bitterly accused feminists working in NGOs and with the state of having sold out. Women from NGOs, still exhausted from the intensity of their work on the UN summits and justifiably proud of the significant achievements of the women's movement in the conference agreements, were dismayed and discouraged by the attacks. However divisive the attacks on NGOs may have been, the conference had the salutary effect of causing many feminist NGOs to take a critical look at the impact on the movement of their relationships with the state.

Mirroring tensions within the Latin American women's movement as a whole, a central strategic tension in many networks in this study revolved around their relationship with the state. The state, of course, is multifaceted, with many internal contradictions. It interfaces at all levels with diverse civil society organizations. In many countries, one arm of the state may commit severe human rights abuses while other state agencies cooperate with civil society organizations to implement programs promoting well-being and human rights (only sometimes including women's rights and sexual and reproductive rights). Colombia's government is a prime example of such contradictions. The military are accused of civil and human rights abuses as they fight the guerrilla forces, whereas entities such as the National Planning Commissions actively seek citizen involvement—with explicit invitations to women's organizations—in decision-making.

Tensions within the women's movement take on different forms in each country and, at times, in each province within a more decentralized country, in response to marked political and institutional variations. Women's organizations may take for granted a high level of cooperation with the state in one part of a country, while organizations in another part may view such cooperation as ethically repugnant. For example, Mexico's National Forum of Women and Population Policy suffered tensions when NGOs based in Mexico City collaborated actively with a municipal administration led by the center-left Democratic Revolutionary Party (PRD), while NGOs based in Chiapas, where the national army and the state government actively repress the Zapatista Army for National Liberation[95] and indigenous movements, could not conceive of cooperating with the state.

While notable cases of overly centralized and/or semiauthoritarian corrupt governments still exist in Latin America, such tendencies coexist with recent reforms that have led to greater decentralization and new public/private partnerships in which the state contracts NGOs to provide services and run programs, generally for low-income sectors. These reforms have coincided with the withdrawal of many international donors from the region, at a time when national philanthropy fails to support political advocacy for social change. As a result, some NGOs have become financially dependent on public contracts as other sources of support dry up, and those NGOs incur much greater costs when they take independent, critical stances toward the state. The greater dependence on the state by some NGOs in the women's rights and reproductive rights movement has exacerbated political tensions within advocacy NGO networks, especially when deliberating between outsider-versus-insider strategies.

Several essays and studies have described the tensions that permeate Latin American women's rights activist groups, which have witnessed the gradual erosion of their institutional autonomy and their critical stance at the same time as they have gained greater public recognition. The groups now engage in dialogue with public entities and coexecute governmental programs. The present challenge is to avoid conceding nonnegotiable principles; however, the limits of such principles often are hazy and ill defined.[96]

The sterilization campaigns carried out by the government of Peru in 1996–1997 provide one example of how NGOs' increased dependence on the state, combined with the political complexities of addressing reproductive rights issues, can paralyze the decision-making of NGO networks. Due to President Alberto Fujimori's strong focus on population control, the Ministry of Health (MOH) implemented an intense target-driven campaign with the goal of sterilizing two million Peruvian women. The MOH gave individual health providers and clinic directors unofficial, but inflexible, monthly quotas for the number of sterilizations—along with both threats and incentives to meet the quotas. Countering the influence of the coercive MOH campaign, large governmental projects supported by multilateral and bilateral donors[97] contracted women's NGOs to carry out programs that were designed to improve quality of care in health services.[98] As a result, some feminist NGOs had a direct financial and political stake in maintaining a positive working relationship with the MOH, leading to severe disagreements in feminist NGO networks on how to address the ministry's human rights abuses in the sterilization campaigns. The NGOs cooperating with the government could argue legitimately that by promoting quality of care, they were defending reproductive rights and users' rights within the MOH system, thus mitigating the negative effects of the sterilization campaigns.

Besides the problem of conflict of interest, disagreements on strategy within the women's movement also stemmed from well-founded fears that denouncing government abuses would play into the hands of ultraconservative forces that were pressuring the MOH to withdraw all access to sterilization.[99] Both these factors led to paralysis in the Peruvian NGO advocacy networks. Even the Peru chapter of CLADEM—the major national women's rights network that eventually documented the human rights abuses in the sterilization campaigns—waited a year after learning about the campaigns to launch its investigation. Peru's National Initiative Group of Women for Equality (Grupo Impulsor) never took a public stand against the campaigns *as a network* although its national assembly, precisely because of concerns about the campaigns, had chosen sexual and reproductive rights as one of two main focuses for monitoring government compliance with the Beijing Platform.[100] In summary, many of the major Peruvian feminist organizations did not take an immediate or firm stand against the sterilization campaigns because some members had a direct financial stake in maintaining good relationships with the government and because they feared that the right wing would take too much advantage of the issue.

CLADEM and one of its members, Centro de la Mujer Peruana Flora Tristán, took action to document and publicize the human rights abuses, and took most of the public heat when the media publicized their study in January 1998. Conservative forces took advantage of the situation, as was feared. U.S. Congressman Chris Smith (R-NJ) conducted a fact-finding visit soon after the story broke in the media in January 1998, then introduced a resolution in the U.S. Congress to cut off all USAID support to Peru. The Fujimori government blamed the network NGOs for the scandal's fallout, and both the author of the study and the Flora Tristán NGO suffered harassment and exclusion from government-controlled contracts.[101]

Another element in the Peruvian women's movement's response to this situation sheds light on the way forward when institutionalized networks— for all the reasons discussed earlier—are unable to reach agreement on their public response to an emerging advocacy issue. After the divisive 1996 Latin American Feminist Meeting in Cartagena and partly in response to the divisions within the Peruvian women's movement on collaboration with the government, feminists in Peru established a noninstitutional advocacy network to answer the need for coordinated feminist participation in such debates. Individual women from prominent feminist NGOs, auto-nomous feminists, and a few organizations formed a new informal network called the Mass Women's Movement (Movimiento Amplio de Mujeres— MAM).[102] Unlike the Cartagena movement, this initiative was not explicitly anti-NGO, but arose from the members' recognition that a space independent of the NGOs was needed for feminist advocacy initiatives. In forming MAM, the members hoped that NGO interests would not block the collective participation of feminists in public debates, as had occurred with networks composed of organizational representatives. "It was the NGO women who determined that they needed a political mechanism to cast a broad net for outreach in order to reconstruct the constituency needed to participate in public debates," MAM's Giulia Tamayo noted.[103] Besides CLADEM, MAM was the only Peruvian feminist network that publicly attacked President Fujimori's sterilization cam-paigns, denouncing both the human rights abuses of the sterilization campaigns and the rights-restricting initiatives of the religious conservatives. Possibly, ad hoc "outsider" coalitions of individuals and some organiza-tions—such as MAM in this case in Peru—are better suited than the institu-tional NGO networks to carry out public, high-profile responses when governments abuse rights, or when the debate surrounding an advocacy issue is highly polarized. These situations are apt to be politically and financially risky for NGOs in the current economic context in most Latin American countries.

Several other voices within the Latin American women's movement view insider-outsider strategies as a false dichotomy. They call for joint strategies that would end stalemates between confrontation/independence versus negotiation/dependence.

We have to arrive at a level of maturity in feminism in which the strategy of denouncing abuses goes hand in hand with negotiation, and in which both strategies spring from the same source without conflicts between us. In general, in Latin American countries, there is no negotiation unless it is preceded by denunciation. ... Some organizations are more apt to negotiate. In others, there are groups advocating both paths. Ideally, there would be no "victims"; that is, we should be the ones to plan this dual strategy, and not have it be them [officials, the government] who divide us. It is impossible to say that one of these strategies is better than the other; it all depends on what you achieve with the strategy, so it is very important to respect the distinct achievements of each strategy.[104]

This mature and coordinated team strategy sounds, in theory, like a wonderful idea to resolve this central divisive issue in the Latin American women's movement, but in fact, when organizations take the route of denouncing government abuses, the strategy incurs real costs. Contracts with governments, and bilateral and multilateral projects that require government approval, have become a key source of income for NGOs, and the experience in Peru shows that governments penalize NGOs that take on the denunciatory role. One solution for this win-lose situation would be for donors who are not required to channel grants through government agencies to give special consideration to NGOs that take the political risk of serving as the public, outsider voice of denunciation when a government abuses human rights or fails to live up to its obligations. The other possibility for NGOs committed to the outsider role is to build their capacity to raise funds from sympathetic individuals, both within their countries and internationally.

The Political Risks of Controversy

Focus on sexual and reproductive rights incurs political costs for NGO advocacy networks and their members because the networks are immersed in cultures that are deeply polarized on these issues. The lack of an internationally recognized covenant covering sexual and reproductive rights is merely a symptom of the lack of consensus in most societies on certain key sexual and reproductive rights. Sexual and reproductive rights advocates generally agree in principle that the right to decide "freely and responsibly" on sexuality[105] should include sexual orientation issues. Likewise, most advocates agree that the "basic right of all couples and individuals to decide freely and responsibly the number, spacing, and timing of their children and to have the information and means to do so, and the right to attain the highest standard of sexual and reproductive health"[106] should include access for people of all ages to all available contraceptive methods and safe abortion services. Intense levels of controversy surround these two issues in particular, and the second is most controversial when applied to youth.

Even agreement in principle among advocates, however, does not always translate into willingness to take action. As mentioned above, the more a network expands its social base in a society that is polarized on these issues, the greater the diversity of opinions within the network. Having a list of basic principles to which all network members must adhere may be essential, but the formal unity achieved by the list can mask important differences in the members' willingness to defend the most controversial principles on the list. Such underlying differences usually take the form of disagreements about appropriate strategies for political action. Thus, some networks in this study did not undertake public advocacy for decriminalization of abortion, and until 2000, none had campaigned for abolishing discrimination based on sexual orientation.

One of the largest regional networks, the Latin American and Caribbean Women's Health Network (LACWHN), confronted the disagreements within the women's movement by setting a firm policy that prevents disagreement among board of director members about defending more controversial sexual and reproductive rights issues.

When we talk about topics such as sexual orientation and decriminalization of abortion, undoubtedly there will be many groups who prefer to stay in the rear-guard. ... Our directors, before they are elected, know that we are going to work on all "feminist health issues," including those of sexual orientation and abortion. That is our bottom line. If they do not accept this, they cannot join the Board.[107]

It is important to note that LACWHN is somewhat protected from potential internal divisions caused by size and diversity of membership because the board, and not an assembly of members, is the group's decision-making body.

When networks do not confront the risk of internal division strategically, they experience conflicts that have the result of limiting the members committed to a controversial issue. In the case of abortion, the coordinator of the Colombian CWNSRR in 1998 explained how a stalemate was resolved following a turning point for the network: an annual assembly in which a strategic planning facilitator helped keep the discussions constructive. Her observations also point to the limitations on statements of principles of unity:

There are diverse opinions within the Network about abortion. Some members have opted for emphasizing quality of care in services, while others work on abortion. It is a kind of division of labor. We have to be pluralist...and arrive at some kind of relationship in which we have basic agreements. They were constructed emotionally, without being clear about their implications. We were very enthusiastic when we first formed the Network, and only a few people wrote the principles. We weren't conscious enough of the difficulties, of the obstacles in our path. The second time that we wrote principles of unity, during the strategic planning exercise, they were developed among those of us who remained [in the network], the most committed. Now we are sure what we want.

Focusing on the more controversial issues in the sexual and reproductive rights field can winnow out the indecisive, often limiting the size of a network. In order to work on issues such as abortion, it helps to have a cohesive group; this is harder to achieve as an NGO network becomes more numerous and diverse.

Besides the risk of dividing a network from within, this study found instances of three other types of political risk incurred by campaigning for decriminalization of abortion: (1) internal division, (2) alienation of the network from potential allies, and (3) "blacklisting,[108] or marginalization by mainstream institutions or governments. In the first kind of risk, the more broad-based the membership of an NGO network member, the more likely that having the NGO's name attached to a controversial initiative on reproductive rights will produce internal conflicts. In the second case, sexual and reproductive rights networks often join broad-based coalitions on important public health or human rights issues, thus expanding their network of allies and contacts. However, their coalition partners may pressure the networks to silence any issues that would be divisive within the coalition. Those working on safe motherhood coalitions to lower maternal mortality know that some organizations in these coalitions are not receptive when other members advocate focusing on the lack of safe abortion services as a factor in mortality. In the citizen's peace movement in Colombia, uniting the women's networks, the human rights movement, and the Catholic Church, coalition partners pressured the CWNSRR to downplay the issue of abortion.

The third type of political risk is also common. Networks or NGOs that are identified with abortion or other controversial issues (such as the sterilization controversies in Peru) might find themselves excluded from certain invitation lists, not considered as speakers at conferences, effectively barred from bidding on government contracts, and, in general, considered as *persona non grata* in any venue where the Catholic Church has influence.

Perceptions of political risk have interfered with strategic decisions and internal divisions in the CWNSRR network. Tensions over abortion-related strategies kept the network from exercising leadership on that issue throughout most of its existence. A national assembly early in the network's life decided on the first "principles of unity," including defense of the right to safe abortion. This did not resolve tensions around the issue, which erupted soon afterward when the NGO in charge of communications for the network omitted all mention of abortion from a published communiqué on maternal mortality on May 28, the International Day for Women's Health. While the anger of the other network members was understandable, it is instructive to consider that the offending NGO was closely linked with a grassroots women's network whose membership was divided on the issue of abortion.

In discussions after this incident, the NGO that issued the communiqué said the disagreement was on strategy, and that the network needed first to gain respect and legitimacy among a wide array of social actors before tackling the abortion issue. They argued that too much focus on abortion would cut off channels of dialogue before they had even opened. This argument represents a universal theme of strategy debates in the advocacy networks in this study. In the author's experience, the most common reason given by feminist NGOs for not addressing the problem of unsafe abortion directly is that they need to gain legitimacy and a broad base of support *before* addressing the issue. While in many instances, especially early in the public life of an NGO or network, valid strategic reasons exist to address broader, related reproductive or civil rights first, this reasoning also has become a perennial excuse. Many NGOs or networks never decide that the time is ripe, whether due to division within their membership or to other political costs of taking on the issue.

Many networks reported stalemated discussions between the more "radical" or "activist" and the more "cautious" members of the network in discussions about strategy on abortion in particular, with mutual hard feelings and blame on both sides. The all-too-common judgment that the more cautious organizations have been "co-opted" poses an obstacle in dealing constructively with organizations' legitimate concern for their own well-being. The underlying challenge is how to collaborate on advocacy for sexual and reproductive rights while balancing three important considerations: the bottom-line principle of defense of rights, the goal of expanding a network's social base, and organizational mandate to do more good than harm to the NGO members of the network. How can one tell when postponing work on access to safe abortions is a valid strategic plan and when is it a perennial excuse? A network cannot ignore the real political costs that organizations incur when they espouse these more controversial reproductive rights. NGO members that suffer unacceptable political costs because of network initiatives, costs such as loss of political legitimacy, damaged relationships with important institutional partners, or loss of important sources of funding may either become weaker institutions or drop out. When members are weakened, the network suffers, because it is only as strong as its members.

NGOs' fears of their inability to withstand political costs—their perception of their own weakness and lack of legitimacy—underlie the overly sequential strategic thinking that leads to permanent inaction on controversial issues. To combat these fears, many NGO advocacy networks adopt strategies that offset the political and financial risks incurred by working on issues such as abortion. These strategies strengthen the member groups by expanding their social bases and building up their political capital in other ways, without postponing their public advocacy for access to safe abortion services. The most common strategy is to address simultaneously other less controversial, but related, issues that bring the network into positive relationships with a broad network of allies. Sometimes, these related issues provide a lead-in to the more controversial issues. Ideally, the NGOs or networks find opportunities in these broader alliances to educate other sectors on sexual and reproductive rights issues.

For example, advocates within safe motherhood initiatives can broach the issue of unsafe abortion as a major cause of maternal mortality. In Colombia, the CWNSSR used the issue of sexual violence as the center of its annual campaign, realizing that the campaign could also serve to soften public opinion to the idea of legalizing abortion in cases of rape and incest. In several countries, highly publicized cases of sexual violence (Paulina in Mexico, Alba Lucia in Colombia) have indeed served to expand the media's sympathetic coverage of pro-choice points of view. The NGOs in the Catholics for the Right to Decide network typically join the social justice organizations of the progressive Catholic Church, where they give workshops and distribute their literature, thus working for social justice, allying themselves with broader efforts for church reform, and legitimizing themselves as Catholics.[109] Also in Mexico, La Alianza—a five-NGO consortium working to build a pro-choice movement—has catalyzed a broad-based citizen's campaign[110] for those civil rights and liberties, such as the right to freedom of religion, that form the foundation for sexual and reproductive rights.[111] The main slogan of the campaign is, "Respect for others' decisions is the foundation of civilization and liberty."

This discussion has analyzed how addressing the controversial aspects of sexual and reproductive rights involves trade-offs between defense of those rights and NGO members' institutional interests. Dependence on state funding of some network members causes pronounced differences of opinion on strategy. In these networks, the successful political strategies that mitigate this trade-off and enable advocacy have involved broadening of the political focus in new alliances, making the network less politically vulnerable.

In summary, the juggling of fidelity to political principles and expansion of one's base of political and financial support leads to a constant search for equilibrium in the NGO networks in this field. The political inertia caused by diverse institutional interests leads to the hypothesis that organizational networks often are not an appropriate mechanism for advocacy strategies related to politically controversial issues that require a rapid public response—strategies that demand agile and independent responses to unexpected situations.[112] The following section contains more reflection on this topic, suggesting how advocacy networks could realize their full political potential.

THE WAY FORWARD

Based on the rich data from NGO advocacy networks, this concluding section puts forward hypotheses about factors and strategies that facilitate NGO network advocacy, and about the tasks and objectives that organizational networks are best suited to undertake.

Evidence from this study indicates that *advocacy by NGO networks can be timely and effective for issues on which wide consensus exists* within the networks. For example, campaigns and political movements related to violence against women, sometimes including sexual violence, seem to attain a high level of political consensus among a broad range of institutions, thus enabling the network to exert effective pressure for policy change. In such cases, a coordinator or designated spokesperson is empowered to make public declarations and act on behalf of network members without engaging in time-consuming and logistically demanding consultations on strategy and on the wording of public pronouncements.

The data on network governance clearly indicates that establishing clear rules on membership, decision-making, financial accountability, and rotation of leadership greatly facilitates NGO network functioning. Networks who attempted to operate by consensus became "entangled" in their decisions on advocacy strategy.

Workshops for internal dialogue and training on the issues can help to produce the needed agreement on basic political principles and strategies. Internal discussions through special workshops and at annual national meetings educated members on controversial sexual and reproductive rights issues and helped them to engage in values clarification through dialogue. For example, Chile's Open Forum for Reproductive and Sexual Health and Rights used training workshops as an effective means of orienting new members to the political framework and agreements forged within the network.

The Forum and others understood that building political agreement among increasingly diverse members is an ongoing activity and a relative concept. If the network is successful in expanding its constituencies, it might never achieve one hundred percent consensus among the members on certain crucial issues. *Many of these networks also benefited from tolerating different levels of risk-taking among their members,* with the understanding that not all public communications strategies are appropriate in varied provincial locales. However, determining when a chapter's strategy does not adhere to the founding principles of the network, and when the chapter is on the same path as the whole network, but at an earlier stage, is a complex exercise and the topic of heated debates in many of these networks.

Provincial level work enjoys some clear advantages. Several provincial NGO network chapters clearly attained greater achievements than those at the national level. Even though the provincial NGOs may be smaller, poorer, and less technically savvy than their sister groups in the capital, this study suggests that they have two advantages. The provincial chapters of a national network are better able to work out internal differences in face-to-face meetings, thus overcoming the logistical difficulties of making decisions on a national level. In Colombia, Peru, and Chile, provincial network chapters have been much more successful than capital-based chapters in establishing dialogue with policymakers that resulted in changes in policies and programs.[113] Possibly, in the less populous venue of provinces, where there are multiple ties among diverse professionals and organizations, it is easier and less time consuming for provincial NGOs to activate their social and political networks among local elites and in local centers of power. Furthermore, in all three countries, the provincial chapters have had better access to the local media, an exposure that increases their potential to influence local public opinion. As one member of Peru's post-Beijing group remarked, "The provinces and Lima have different dynamics; we have a much harder time being heard here in Lima."

Investment in training and internal dialogue not only helps network members to forge agreements on political strategy, but also to advance the important long-term goal of building the members' capacity to address advocacy issues appropriately and professionally with a variety of audiences. NGO advocacy networks seem to be well-suited to this strategy, which is of clear benefit to the members. In this study, training opportunities were one of the most-mentioned benefits of belonging to an advocacy network. Training interventions thus served the dual purpose of forging cohesion among older and newer networks members, and building advocacy capacity in a variety of ways.

The *networks also achieved the goal of capacity-building in advocacy through projects that funded provincial chapters' activities in network-wide initiatives;* in this study the most compelling evidence on capacity-building comes from interviews and reports about such initiatives, which have the added advantage of corresponding to the project-based logic of donor agencies. For example, Peru's post-Beijing National Initiative Group of Women for Equality's (Grupo Impulsor) national monitoring effort centered on compliance with quotas for women in electoral slates and on sexual and reproductive rights. Even though the national network was unable to respond adequately to the reproductive rights abuses in government sterilization campaigns, this initiative energized, trained, and empowered many provincial groups. According to the testimony of provincial leaders,[114] the monitoring gave them an effective new way to exercise citizenship and demand accountability from local authorities, an advocacy skill that will serve them for multiple purposes into the future.

One prominent example of such beneficial national initiatives emerged from this study. *Support for national consultation processes before and after UN conferences* re-energized national women's movements and created new networks. In the countries in this study, the NGO members of national networks—especially the small and provincial groups—had a very positive view of the training sessions and national meetings that took place before and after the UN conferences in the mid-1990s. The study also documents the negative consequences for a national network when funding disappears after the UN summit is over. Without adequate follow-up funding, the diverse range of women's perspectives—especially from low-income, provincial, and/or rural women—are not represented in a network's decision-making structures.

As noted earlier, advocacy on controversial issues such as abortion can cause internal divisions, loss of alliances, loss of political influence, and loss of financial support. This study demonstrates how some NGO networks have counteracted these risks to the institutional interests of members. *NGO networks have joined broader alliances and undertaken significant initiatives on less controversial issues.* These alliances and initiatives help unite network members, build internal trust and relationships, and they provide opportunities to educate the broad alliance members on the core issues of the advocacy network. Finally, they help to ensure that a network and its members do not lose important political contacts and bases of support as they move forward on more controversial issues.

Finally, the experience from Peru with MAM—the ad hoc feminist coalition that denounced the sterilization campaigns—suggests that similar *ad hoc coalitions, arising from multiple overlapping institutional and informal networks, may be the most useful vehicle for engaging in public debate on controversial emerging issues* that could incur political costs for NGOs. Although institutionalized NGO advocacy networks may not be well-suited for these rapid responses to political crises, especially when confrontation with government is involved, they can *serve an important function as a launching pad for organizing these impromptu political initiatives,* which often draw on selected members of more than one advocacy network.

However, some participants in MAM in Peru have pointed out that as the life of their ad hoc coalition continues, MAM has begun to suffer from some of the same obstacles to decision-making experienced in the more institutionalized NGO networks. *Although ad hoc coalitions may achieve notable political successes, their ability to act decisively in politically risky situations may actually depend on having a short life and informal character.* If so, then the longer such a coalition stays alive, the more it will fall prey to the same institutional barriers noted in this study.[115]

Evidence from the study noted that *access to the Internet* is a facilitating factor for networks, reducing the cost of communications as access expands to the provincial and less-developed regions of Latin American countries. With regard to forming ad hoc coalitions, the Internet has increased exponentially the speed at which these can be formed. However, many women in rural areas or with lower educational levels still face considerable barriers to engagement in Internet-based networks or coalitions.

Given that the main obstacles to consensus on highly visible strategies arise from the political and financial risks incurred by the networks' NGO members, it seems that *NGO networks are ideally suited for less visible advocacy strategies,* such as private policy dialogue with decision-makers, when the issues are highly controversial. The findings from this study should lead to a rethinking of many activists' unspoken assumption that a public pronouncement on breaking news is the most important bottom-line activity for an advocacy network. While the study suggests some strategies for mitigating those risks, an NGO network clearly is a cumbersome vehicle for highly public, controversial advocacy strategies. On the other hand, NGO network members could be deployed to great advantage to engage in private dialogue and negotiations with each one's contacts among the political and media elites, thus realizing the networks' potential for complementary and synergistic actions.

In summary, NGO advocacy networks may be best suited to pursue longer-term objectives related to increasing members' advocacy capacity and expanding their social base, while engaging in the painstaking and often conflictual process of building agreement on political objectives and strategies among diverse organizations. However, the investment in time and resources in advocacy networks is only justified if they produce better results in policy change than NGOs working on their own. Although these networks may be limited in their ability to respond agilely on emerging controversial issues, this study suggests that once the members of a network have reached agreement about political strategies and have developed mechanisms for rapid response, their potential positive impact on rights-related policies is indeed greater than the sum of the parts.

The areas of achievement in this study, then, point a way forward to realizing this potential. The political and financial risks for NGOs arising from advocacy on the most controversial sexual and reproductive rights issues are a given fact. They will not disappear, and at the moment of writing this conclusion in 2005 they seem to be increasing. Therefore, networks need to take advantage of all the facilitating factors and strategies mentioned above in order to minimize risks and increase results—building closer connections to financial and political elites, joining broader coalitions with related goals, strengthening advocacy work at the provincial and local levels, investing in internal dialogue and training to build agreements and technical expertise, tolerating varying levels of risk-taking among members, and engaging in private, behind-the-scenes policy dialogue. In this way, NGO networks should be enabled to move forward on the most politically risky issues and, at the same time, build capacity among their members and increased legitimacy for the full range of issues in their political agenda.

The main questions that each NGO advocacy network must ask itself have to do with the need to balance the institutional interests of the members with the advocacy goals of the network. How to minimize the political risks, yet still maximize the results of advocacy strategies? How to gain access to, and influence with, political elites without sacrificing the more controversial basic commitments to women's rights and sexual and reproductive rights? How to expand the membership and social base of a network without watering down these commitments?

Other important questions relate to the organizational means to these ends: How to be less "entangled" when deciding on strategies? How to organize decision-making efficiently and democratically? How to become less financially dependent on foreign donors and/or the government? Whether and how to expand and diversify in membership? How to involve low-income women, rural women, provincial women, women from ethnic minorities, and women from other marginalized sectors in meaningful ways?

Each network makes choices in responding to these questions, sometimes implicitly, or without foreseeing their consequences. The author hopes that this analysis of the experiences of NGO advocacy networks in Latin America may help similar networks make conscious, well-informed decisions on these important questions.[116]

APPENDIX A: NETWORKS INTERVIEWED FOR THIS STUDY AND SOURCES OF INFORMATION

Some networks for which information is incomplete are included in this list because the author took advantage of unforeseen opportunities to interview activists from these networks during the data collection phase, from 1998 through 2000.

National Networks

Colombian Women's Network for Sexual and Reproductive Rights— CWNSRR (Red Colombiana de Mujeres por los Derechos Sexuales y Reproductivos) was founded in 1992 at a national meeting and has six city chapters. Sources of data: group interviews by the author in Bogotá, Cali, and Medellín; reports to the Ford Foundation; and internal CWNSRR documents.

National Women's Network, Colombia (Red Nacional de Mujeres) was formed in 1991 to unify women's organizations' input into the Constitutional Assembly. The network now includes fourteen provincial networks and eighty organizations. The current focal point is the Corporación Sisma Mujer (SISMA Women's Corporation) in Bogotá. Sources of data: a group interview in Bogotá and personal correspondence with Beatriz Quintero.[117]

National Initiative Group of Women for Equality, Peru (Grupo Impulsor Nacional Mujeres por la Igualdad), a Lima-based group of NGOs formed before the Beijing Conference, has expanded in numbers since 1995 to monitor compliance with the Beijing Plan of Action. The group coordinates actions with an average of ten NGOs in each region of the country. Sources of data: a group interview in Lima and the author's attendance at a national meeting with representatives from all of the active provinces. A Peruvian NGO, CESIP (Center for Social Studies and Publications), has coordinated the group since its inception. Web site: http://www.cesip.org.pe.

Open Forum for Reproductive and Sexual Health and Rights-Chile (Red de Salud y Derechos Sexuales y Reproductivos-Chile) (now called Health Forum or Foro Salud). Founded in 1989, this NGO network now has six provincial subnetworks and fifty-two member organizations. Sources of data: two group interviews in 1998–1999, reports to the Ford Foundation, and publications. Web site: www.forosalud.cl/acerca.html.

Post-Beijing Initiative Group, Chile (Grupo Iniciativa de Mujeres) is a Santiago-based group of NGOs formed before the Beijing Conference and expanded since 1995 to promote and monitor compliance with the Beijing Plan of Action. Sources of data: interviews with ISIS Internacional and Teresa Valdés of FLACSO and publications of the Group. Web site: http://www.flacso.cl. Go to Investigaciones, Estudios de Género, then "Ciudadanía y Control Ciudadano."

Network against Violence against Women, Chile (Red contra Violencia contra las Mujeres). Sources of data: partial information only, from interview with Mireya Zuleta, Casa de la Mujer de Valparaiso, and Isabel Duque of ISIS Internacional.

The National Forum of Women and Population Policy, México (Foro Nacional de Mujeres y Políticas de Población) was created in 1993 in preparation for ICPD and now monitors and promotes governmental compliance with the ICPD Programme of Action. The Forum includes eighty Mexican women's organizations and academic institutions from eighteen of the thirty-one Mexican states. Sources of data: incomplete information from interview with one of the coordinators and Forum documents. Web site: http://www.laneta.apc.org/foropob/.

Community Network for Prevention of HIV/ AIDS (Chile) is an NGO network founded in 1991 that has a history of divisions and conflicts. Sources of data: partial information only from interview with ex-member, and two papers about the network.

Regional Networks

Catholics for the Right to Decide in Latin America (Católicas por el Derecho a Decidir, Latinoamérica—CDD/LA) is a network of seven sister organizations with the same name in Mexico, Colombia, Bolivia, Chile, Argentina, and Brazil. The network promotes women's rights and sexual and reproductive rights from a Catholic perspective through research, education, and advocacy. The CDDs in Latin America participate with the U.S.-based Catholics for a Free Choice (CFFC) in various global activities and exchanges. Web site: http://www.catolicasporelderechoadecidir.org/.

ISIS Internacional (Chile) is a women's information and communication service founded in 1974. Two other sister organizations named ISIS were founded in the Philippines and Uganda. ISIS promotes the formation of communications networks, both global and regional. Sources of data: group interview providing information on several networks and observations on networks in general. Web site: http://www.isis.cl/.

Latin American and Caribbean Committee for the Defense of Women's Rights (Comité de América Latina y el Caribe para la Defensa de los Derechos de la Mujer—CLADEM) was founded in 1987 and now has seventeen country groups or active contacts (*enlaces*). Its mission is to develop and disseminate legal research, training, jurisprudence, campaigns, and proposals to defend women's rights. Web site: http:// www.cladem.org/.

Latin American and Caribbean Women's Health Network—LACWHN (Red de Salud de Mujeres Latinoamericanos y del Caribe—RSMLAC) was created in 1984 in the First Regional Meeting on Women's Health in Tenza, Colombia. This large network is composed of organizations and individuals, with publications, training programs, and activist campaigns in favor of women's health and rights. The regional office is in Santiago, Chile. Web site: http://www.reddesalud.org/.

Latin American and Caribbean Feminist Network against Domestic and Sexual Violence (Red Feminista Latinoamericano y del Caribe contra la Violencia Doméstica y Sexual). Sources of data: partial information only from ISIS Internacional interview and from web site, http://www.isis.cl/redes/redfeminista.htm.

NOTES

1. Beatriz Quintero, the National Women's Network, Colombia.

2. This paper contains some information updated in 2002.

3. See Appendix A for a list and description of the networks included in this study. The national networks included in this study are in Colombia, Peru, Chile, and Mexico.

4. Oré Aguilar 1999, 2.

5. The Pathfinder Fund has since changed its name to Pathfinder International. During an internal reorganization, Pathfinder eliminated the Women's Programs Division in 1986.

6. The sample for this study is opportunistic, based on organizations the author worked with or had access to during the data collection phase in 1998–2000. Updated information from 2002 comes partly from e-mails exchanged with those interviewed at the earlier time. In addition, the author worked as a senior consultant for Catholics for Free Choice during 2001–2005, working closely with members of the Católicas por el Derecho a Decidir (CDD) network. This work has put her in touch with current developments in the regional networks and some of the country networks. Some information from the CDD network was added in 2002.

7. The countries discussed in this article differ in nomenclature for their political-geographical subdivisions. Some countries have regions and provinces within regions, while others have states or departments. To avoid confusion, I use the term "provinces" throughout to refer to the geopolitical divisions of a country outside the capital.

8. The exceptions to this rule are foundations such as the Global Fund for Women, which are set up explicitly as small grants programs.

9. See Keck and Sikkink 1998 for details.

10. Keck and Sikkink 1998, 168–169.

11. In "Thoughts on Distinctive Logics of Transnational Feminism," Alvarez argues that transnational feminist activism obeys two distinct logics: the transnational advocacy logic attempts "to expand formal rights or influence public policy," as in the advocacy surrounding the UN conferences, while the "logic of mutual solidarity and identity" aims mainly to "(re)construct and, or reaffirm subaltern political identities and to establish strategic and personal bonds of solidarity with others who share particular values (for example feminist ideals), or traits (for example lesbians)."

12. The NGO (nongovernmental organization) Forum is the civil society conference that parallels an official UN conference composed of government delegations. Many of the UN conferences have had NGO Forums with substantial representation from NGOs.

13. The literature on the role of NGO networks in the Cairo and Beijing UN conferences in particular is vast, and only a handful of sources that provide summaries are included in the references (Gruskin 1995; Dunlop, Kyte, and MacDonald 1996; Girard 1999; Population Council and Population Reference Bureau 1999). For past and current information on follow-up actions from these conferences, the web sites of the following organizations contain useful articles, summaries, and access to other publications: WomenWatch (http://www.un.org/womenwatch); the Women's Environment and Development Organization (WEDO); the Center for Reproductive Rights; the International Women's Health Coalition; ISIS Internacional; the Latin American and Caribbean Women's Health Network; the Latin American and Caribbean Committee for the Defense of Women's Rights (CLADEM—Comité de América Latina y el Caribe para la Defensa de los Derechos de la Mujer); the United Nations Fund for Population Activities (UNFPA); and the United Nations Development Fund for Women (UNIFEM).

14. See Center for Reproductive Rights and DEMUS (Estudio para la Defensa de los Derechos de la Mujer—Office for the Defense of Women's Rights) 2001, 80–88, for a full discussion of reproductive rights trends in the region. The full text of the Inter-American Convention on the Prevention, Punishment, and Eradication of Violence against Women ("Convention of Belém Do Pará," ratified in 1994); accessed on October 2005: http://www.oas.org/juridico/english/sigs/a-61.html.

15. Regional analyses from CLADEM's November 2001 seminar on sexual and reproductive rights; accessed in 2002 on the web site of the Campaign to Promote an Inter-American Sexual and Reproductive Rights Convention: http://www.convencion.org.uy, but no longer available; see latest regional analysis for 2003 under "documentos."

16. UNAIDS, Barcelona Presskit, 2002, 35. This is no longer available on the Web site.

17. CLADEM 2001, op. cit.

18. Personal communications in 2002 with Astrid Bant of the International Women's Health Coalition, Luisa Cabal of the Center for Reproductive Rights, Susana Chiarotti of CLADEM, Virginia Chambers of IPAS, Frances Kissling of Catholics for Free Choice (USA), and Gaby Oré Aguilar of the Ford Foundation.

19. As of 2006, the following section is somewhat outdated. In 2002, Mexico was the exception to this trend, and as of January 2006, abortion law reform efforts are in

process in Colombia and Argentina. A 2004 effort in Uruguay almost gained enough support to win.

20. The Global Gag Rule prohibits organizations that receive U.S. foreign aid from engaging in advocacy for legal abortion and from providing legal abortion services or referrals for legal abortions; see the web site of the Center for Reproductive Rights for more information about the Global Gag Rule, accessed on October 2005: http://www.reproductiverights.org/hill_int_ggr.html.

21. The most notable recent achievements include the success of the Brazilian HIV/AIDS movement in securing access to medicines, approval for and availability of emergency contraception in several countries, and expansion of the grounds for legal abortion in some Mexican states.

22. With their ability to achieve impact on the abortion issue stalled, the NGO networks and their members tend to judge the relative success of any advocacy or communications strategy by the number of people or organizations involved in the action, by direct feedback from participants in events, and by the amount of media coverage. While these are important intermediate indicators, over the long run a relative lack of continuing policy impact might erode the support of the few donors still active in Latin America with a focus on reproductive rights.

23. See the web site http://www.convencion.org.uy/default. htm for a description of the campaign and a list of the sponsoring networks and organizations.

24. Information on the Alliance comes from internal documents.

25. The Erik E. and Edith H. Bergstrom Foundation and Ipas have supported many of these efforts.

26. See all writings listed in references by Sonia Alvarez, Maruja Barrig, and Roberto P. Korzeniewicz and William C. Smith.

27. Barrig, De Cal y Arena, 1997.

28. In 1992, only 5.5 percent of Colombian NGOs reported receiving aid from foreign governments, while 18 percent report support from international and national foundations (Vargas et al. 1992, 61–62). Some 62 percent of revenues were self-generated. The figures for Peru are similar, with 68 percent of self-generated income, while 22 percent of nonprofit income comes from international donors and lenders (Sanborn 2000, 6).

29. Barrig, La Larga Marcha, 1997.

30. For a fuller discussion of recent trends in the philanthropic sector in Latin America, see Sanborn 2000 and the Latin American section of Salamon et al. 1999.

31. Sanborn 2000, 6.

32. This statement does not pertain to organizations advocating civil and sexual rights for lesbians and gay men. These organizations usually are composed of volunteer activists. A small number of U.S. foundations provide general support in Latin America for women's rights and reproductive rights advocacy, and several of these foundations explicitly focus on efforts to legalize abortion. The author's conversations with NGOs from several different Latin American countries support Sanborn's finding that most international and national donors support projects that directly benefit low-income and vulnerable sectors, as opposed to advocacy projects that aim to influence political and financial elites.

33. Wisely 1990, 57.

34. In part, this is because the activists in these movements often come from the ranks of the left or progressive movements, which had been weakened greatly in most countries in 2002 at the time of writing this article. However, in 2006, four years after completing this article, the panorama looks quite different, with several left-of-center governments in Latin America. The strong connection of many members of the Brazilian feminist movement with the leftist, but very powerful, Workers' Party (Partido dos Trabalhadores—PT) of President Luiz Inácio da Silva (Lula) has helped to bring many feminists into positions of local or national authority.

35. Knoke 1990, 5–6. Knoke describes persuasive power: "[It] relies only on the informational content of messages, with no ability to invoke sanctions for refusal to comply." Persuasive power cannot rely on domination (such as the "power to control the behavior of another by offering or withholding some benefit or harm") but does rely on influence (such as the transmission of information that alters another's behavior through communication from a source viewed as "legitimate" and authoritative). "Coercive power" has domination, but no influence, while "authoritative power" has both.

36. Wisely 1990, 65.

37. Korzeniewicz, *Civil Society Networks*, 2001, 16.

38. A leader from the Open Forum for Reproductive and Sexual Health and Rights—Chile.

39. An interesting discussion of the pros and cons of various strategies was published by the Ford Foundation following a meeting of grantees of the Sexual and Reproductive Health Program in the Andean and Southern Cone Region (Ford Foundation and ICMER 1999).

40. Some of the content of this section has been updated to include the author's personal knowledge of strategies initiated during the 2000–2002 period.

41. See the web site of the Latin American and Caribbean Women's Health Network (RSMLAC) under "Campaigns" for information on the current focus of each of these days of action; accessed in October 2005: http://www.reddesalud.org/english.

42. The author had no opportunity to update this observation to 2005 in light of recent trends in NGO network advocacy.

43. Paulo Freire's classic work (1986 [1970]) explains how his ideas transformed "popular education" in Brazil by combining a new method of teaching reading with consciousness raising (*conscientização*) techniques. Freire and other Brazilian exiles disseminated these practices throughout Latin America and among progressive community development groups worldwide. The framework of *conscientização* was adopted by the women's movement and has formed the theoretical and methodological basis for training by women's groups for such a long time that many no longer acknowledge or even realize its origins.

44. In participatory methods, the professionals "own" the resulting plans for improvement, yielding much better results when such plans are implemented. These methods also provide NGOs with an insider's view of the stresses faced by overworked, underpaid health professionals in the public sector. The resulting empathy has enabled these NGOs to be effective brokers in promoting dialogue between the health sector and community organizations. Most of the networks in

this study were able to give examples of such mediation; see Chapter 3 for an in-depth case study of Consorcio Mujer (Women's Consortium) in Peru, an alliance of five NGOs that used this strategy combined with training of women's organizations to promote the rights of users of health services.

45. Many of the networks in this study receive a significant proportion of their funds from U.S. donors, which somewhat restricts their ability to engage in these campaigns because of U.S. IRS restrictions on lobbying by nonprofit organizations. NGOs that receive general support from European donors can lobby, but European support is decreasing in the region. The Global Gag Rule was not in effect at the time of this study but poses another significant obstacle at present (2005).

46. CLADEM 2001 op. cit.; information on the campaign in Chile from personal communication of the author with Lidia Casas and Dr. Soledad Diaz of the Instituto Chileno de Medecina Reproductiva (ICMER) in October 2001, and with Claudia Dides of FLACSO in Chile in May 2002; information on the coalition in Colombia came from Janneth Lozano of Católicas por el Derecho a Decidir in Colombia and Cecilia Barraza from Sisma Mujer.

47. A fuller discussion of some lessons from experience in the Peruvian multisectoral committee is in Chapter 3 on Consorcio Mujer and in Consorcio Mujer 2000.

48. On the Alba Lucia case, see discussions and box in the section below on Managing Growth and Diversity. The highly publicized case of Paulina is documented in a book by Elena Poniatowska, *Las mil y una ... la herida de Paulina*, Mexico City: Plaza y Janés, 2000; a thirteen-year-old girl in Baja California who had been raped was denied a legal abortion in her local hospital through delay tactics and harassment. Marta Lamas wrote a brief description of the case in her recent book, *Política y Reproducción Aborto: La Frontera del Derecho a Decidir*, Barcelona and Mexico City: Plaza y Janés, 2001, 153–160.

49. Barrig, *Relatoría General*, 1999, 12.

50. Medillin chapter, CWNSRR.

51. Much of the political science literature relevant to national NGO advocacy networks focuses on political coalitions.

52. Anderson and Frasca 1993 and Swedish International Development Agency 2000 are the main examples the author has found from Latin America that specifically focus on internal governance. The various writings of Maruja Barrig and Sonia Alvarez tend to focus more on tensions within the women's movement and on relations between the women's movement and the state. For literature on internal tensions in the transnational advocacy networks, see Keck and Sikkink 1998 and Korzeniewicz and Smith 2001.

53. Hula 1999; Kingslow Associates 1998; Rose 2000.

54. Korzeniewicz and Smith 2001, 6.

55. The regional networks CLADEM and Católicas por el Derecho a Decidir, Latinoamérica consciously limit growth, as do the two post–Beijing networks in Peru and Chile. LACWHN, on the other hand, is a much larger network and aims to expand.

56. Beatriz Quintero, National Women's Network, Columbia.

57. Knoke 1990, 62–64 summarizes the influential theories of economist Mancur Olson, *The Logic of Collective Action*, Cambridge, MA: Harvard University Press, 1965, about the "free rider" problem. Olson argued that incentives were

insufficient for collective action to produce public goods such as environmental protection and nuclear disarmament. Knoke cites the numerous studies that point out the complexity of people's motivations for becoming politically engaged in advocacy for public goods.

58. Elizabeth Jelin makes this point about the lack of financial accountability of the NGO sector in general in "Toward a Culture of Participation and Citizenship," in Alvarez, Dagnino, and Escobar 1998, 412.

59. A full description of the decision-making and authority structure of the major regional networks in the study is available from the author. This was part of the first draft of the study, which was distributed in Spanish to all the networks in the study.

60. The post–Beijing Grupo Impulsor (National Initiative Group of Women for Equality) in Peru. This was true of the Latin American and Caribbean Women's Health Network (LACWHN) until early 2002, when a new coordinator from Colombia took over.

61. S. Chiarotti, CLADEM.

62. ISIS International group interview.

63. The literature on this subject is extensive, much of it inspired by the seminal work by Carol Gilligan, *In a Different Voice: Psychological Theory and Women's Development*, Cambridge, MA: Harvard University Press, 1982 and 1993.

64. ISIS interview, op. cit. (see note 63).

65. T. Valdes, Post–Beijing Initiative Group, Chile.

66. ISIS International group interview.

67. Coordinator of Cali Chapter, CWNSRR at the time of the interviews in 1999.

68. Brown and Fox 1998, 18–20.

69. The 16 Days of Activism against Gender Violence is an international campaign originating from the first Women's Global Leadership Institute, sponsored by the Center for Women's Global Leadership in 1991. Participants chose the dates between November 25, International Day against Violence against Women, and December 10, International Human Rights Day, in order to make a symbolic linkage of violence against women and human rights and to emphasize that such violence is a violation of human rights. More information is available from the web site of the Center for Women's Global Leadership; accessed in October 2005: http://www.cwgl.rutgers.edu/16days/home.html.

70. Isabel Duque, network coordinator at the time of the interviews in 2000.

71. For purposes of this article, "membership" involves full entitlement in decision-making and in receiving the benefits accruing to members, while the "social base" of the network is a more general concept that refers to the broader set of social actors (entities and individuals) with whom the network interacts and who can be counted on to support at least some of the network's initiatives. Increases in membership result from either an invitation by the network or an application by those interested in joining, with varying degrees of formality in the process. Increases in the social base usually result from expanded outreach through coalition building, training/education, and communications.

72. This observation is based on the author's personal experience in working on strategic planning with NGOs in Latin America and on some statements in the interviews in this study.

73. T. Valdes, Initiative Group, Chile, December 1998. Both the Colombian National Women's Network and the Chilean Post–Beijing Initiative Group have received some support from international donors since the 1998 interviews.

74. Mische and Pattison 2000, 169; Watts 1996.

75. Rose 2000; Kingslow Associates 1998.

76. CWNSRR, Cali Chapter, Group interview.

77. Conversations with the author by women's NGO coalition leaders in Peru and Mexico in 2002. The coalitions that were the subject of these conversations are not included in this study.

78. Foweraker 1995; Hula 1999; Mische and Pattison 2000; Rose 2000; Watts 1996.

79. Mische and Pattison 2000, 164.

80. Watts 1996, 43.

81. Rose 2000, 143.

82. The terms "grassroots," "community-based," and "low-income" are used somewhat interchangeably in the following section as translations for the ubiquitous adjective in Spanish: "popular."

83. The divisions between the low-income women's organizations and the feminist NGOs have often erupted into the public eye, and have been written about extensively by Latin American feminists, including Virginia Vargas, Maruja Barrig, and Sonia Alvarez.

84. Kingslow Associates 1998, 34–36.

85. Of the countries included in this study, Colombia is an exception to this generalization. Throughout much of Colombia's history, the urban centers of Cali and Medellín have been strong centers of political and economic power. In the Colombian network, therefore, the Cali and Medellín chapters are not relatively disadvantaged. To the contrary, they exercised much stronger national leadership within the network than the Bogotá chapter, which tended to be weak and divided.

86. The two post–Beijing groups (Peru and Chile) and CLADEM in Peru belong to the latter group, while the most institutionalized examples of the former are the Open Forum in Chile, the Colombian Sexual and Reproductive Rights Network (CWNSRR), and the National Forum of Women and Population Policy in Mexico. Some of the less-institutionalized networks, such as the National Women's Network in Colombia, were still in the process of developing clear decision rules on this issue at the time of the interviews in 1998.

87. Rich 1996, 6–7.

88. "Voluntary motherhood" emphasizes the idea that no woman with an unplanned pregnancy should be forced to be a mother if she is unwilling to be one. The phrase refers to the "basic right of all couples and individuals to decide freely and responsibly the number, spacing, and timing of their children, and to have the information and means to do so"; see language in ICPD Programme of Action, Chapter 7.

89. The information on the National Women's Network reflects the situation at the time of the interview with Beatriz Quintero and other network members in October 1998. In July 2000, Quintero noted, "The Network has received some resources, and communication has improved greatly. What I said was true at the time, but now [this communication] has generated positive changes and the

Network is more visible" (personal communication to the author). The Network is still mentioned in 2005 communications on Colombian women's movement activities, but the author is no longer in touch with the coordinators to verify its current status.

90. Coordinator of the Open Forum, Chile.

91. CWNSSR, Medellin group interview.

92. This account of events represents the perception of the Network members who were excluded. Tim Frasca and Karen Anderson circulated an unpublished paper in 1993 describing the Network's process.

93. Korzeniewicz and Smith 2001, 4–6.

94. See Alvarez's writings on this topic and Keck and Sikkink 1998, 168–169. Many of the "autonomous" Latin American women's organizations view all collaboration with the state as a compromise of the feminist agenda.

95. The EZLN (Ejército Zapatista de Liberación Nacional—Zapatista Army for National Liberation) is a guerrilla group—closely identified with the indigenous movement—that controls large areas in the highlands of Chiapas.

96. Barrig, *Relatoría General*, 1999, 6; Sonia Alvarez's writings also deal with this topic.

97. Multilateral refers to agencies such as UN agencies and the World Bank, which channel aid from many governments. Bilateral aid is government to government.

98. The Basic Health and Nutrition Project, funded by the World Bank, conducted community-based needs assessments, for which they contracted feminist NGOs. Project 2000, funded by USAID with Pathfinder International, aimed to raise the quality of care and user satisfaction in many services where it intervened. Most notably, Reprosalud, a USAID-funded $19 million project, was awarded in 1994 to one of the largest feminist NGOs in Peru—Movimiento Manuela Ramos—to implement on a massive scale, in low-income provinces, a model community participation program in reproductive health and credit programs for women.

99. See Barrig, *La Persistencia*, 1999, for a fuller discussion of these tensions and the role of Opus Dei in the public controversies about the sterilization campaigns.

100. Grupo Impulsor Nacional 1998. The report from this monitoring describes, but does not highlight, the coercive practices of the sterilization campaigns in one page out of fifty-two pages on sexual and reproductive health. Only two recommendations out of the fifteen presented mention the campaigns, with no corrective action suggested.

101. The home office of attorney Guilia Tamayo of CLADEM, the principal investigator in the study, was broken into, and all of her work-related materials were stolen in October 1998.

102. http://www.apuntes.org/paises/peru/ensayo/mam_agenda.html, accessed on October 31, 2005; contains the political agenda of MAM, developed at a much later date than these events, in 2000.

103. The information on MAM is based on a personal communication to the author by Giulia Tamayo, April 15, 2000.

104. S. Chiarotti, CLADEM.

105. Fourth World Conference on Women, Platform for Action, paragraph 96: "The human rights of women include their right to have control over and decide freely and responsibly on matters related to their sexuality, including sexual and

reproductive health, free of coercion, discrimination, and violence." The full document is available from WomenWatch web site accessed in October 2005: http://www.un.org/womenwatch/daw/beijing/platform/plat1.htm.

106. ICPD Programme of Action Summary, Chapter 7, section A, paragraph 2, quoting "international human rights documents and other relevant UN consensus documents."

107. Amparo Claro, the Coordinator of the LACWHN through much of its early history until 1998.

108. The term "blacklist" is used in its meaning in the United States: a widely circulated list of people who are denied employment because of their political beliefs or activities. The U.S. business sector has employed blacklists to exclude known trade union organizers. The entertainment industry during the McCarthy era in the 1950s excluded people accused of sympathizing with communism. The term *lista negra* has more extreme connotations in Latin America, often meaning a list of people identified for execution or imprisonment by dictatorships or death squads.

109. The church hierarchy typically tries to delegitimize these organizations by saying that they are not true Catholics. In one case in which a Católicas por el Derecho a Decidir (CDD) group successfully educated such allies, more than forty Catholic organizations awarded CDD Mexico the prestigious Don Sergio National Human Rights Prize in 2002 for "defense of women's human rights both within and beyond the Catholic Church."

110. La Ronda Ciudadana (the citizen's round dance) is the name of the campaign, connoting the playful and musical aspects of a circle game or a dance. For more information, see the following web site, in Spanish; accessed in October 2005 at http://www.laronda.org.mx/.

111. This five-organization consortium aims to build a massive pro-choice movement in Mexico, and La Ronda Ciudadana is just one of the strategies adopted. The organizations are Information Group for Reproductive Choice (Grupo de Información sobre Reproducción Elegida—GIRE); Equidad de Género: Ciudadanía, Trabajo y Familia (Gender Equity: Citizenship, Labor and Family); Católicas por el Derecho a Decidir; the Population Council; and Ipas. In the letter of principles, the first principle includes liberty of conscience and liberty of political and religious beliefs, saying, "We demand that others do not impose these beliefs on us, even if they are in the majority."

112. Jael Silliman 1999, 141 makes a similar point with regard to the Green Belt Movement (GBM) in Kenya: "I would go so far as to argue that [resisting institutionalization] has allowed the GBM to act independent of political pressures, as the organization's survival does not rest on donor or government approval, but on its members' tree-planting actions and the ability to galvanize them into political action."

113. These provincial-level successes in policy impact probably depend at least partially on the degree of decentralization in a country. In the study in Chapter 3, provincial organizations in the Consorcio Mujer project in Peru achieved more gains in negotiations with their local health officials than did the three capital-based NGOs, in a situation in which the decentralization structures of the health sector reform had not yet been implemented in Lima.

114. The author heard this testimony at a national meeting of the Grupo Impulsora in Peru 1998.

115. It seems that MAM split into two groups—one called "MAM—The Founding Line" (*Linea Fundacional*) at some point after the events in this study; see Web site accessed January 29, 2006: http://mamfundacional.org/. However, the author was not able to verify this with a MAM participant.

116. The former publication based on this study, published by North-South Center Press, includes an appendix with recommendations for network governance, adapted and expanded from Hord 2002, 55–56.

117. As of October 2005, this network did not have a functioning Web site, but seems to be still active in women's movement initiatives.

3

"LET'S BE CITIZENS, NOT PATIENTS!": PROMOTING PARTNERSHIPS BETWEEN WOMEN'S GROUPS AND HEALTH SERVICES IN PERU

Now we understand that human rights include the right to health. This caused us to think deeply. Why do we let them mistreat us? Why aren't we capable of reacting or asking for what we want. (Member of user committee in Cusco)

What about my rights? Who is going to look out for me when I apply quality principles and they fire me for not meeting my quotas? (Doctor in Piura)

INTRODUCTION

In the traditionally hierarchical context of medical services, both health professionals and users are prisoners of unspoken assumptions and corresponding roles. The shift to a more democratic, horizontal system demands greater consciousness of and respect for users' rights on the part of providers, and both consciousness of rights and the capacity to demand respect for these rights on the part of users. Much effort in the public health and population fields has been devoted to working with reproductive health service providers to improve quality of care and respect for individual rights. Simultaneously, mainly feminist and some community health and development nongovernmental organizations (NGOs) have paid attention to working with users so that they recognize and demand their rights.

Program designers often don't recognize that in order to achieve this shift, an intense process of questioning of assumptions and attitudes on both sides is necessary. At the same time, within the health service, structural measures are necessary, such as changes in evaluation indicators of quality, mechanisms for user feedback and community involvement, and greater quality-related incentives. How can programs help users to construct their identities as citizens with rights so that they demand their rights and recognize violations of rights? How can programs help health providers respect these rights, and be more receptive to power sharing in an egalitarian relationship with users?

This case study of an innovative community participation program in Peru—implemented by a consortium of six feminist organizations called Consorcio Mujer—analyzes the experience of six diverse communities in Peru in which NGOs worked with both providers and users to improve quality of care and respect for users' rights. The sources of data for this study are: (1) reports and documents produced by Consorcio Mujer; (2) the author's personal knowledge of the project as a program officer for the Ford Foundation during the period 1993–1998; and (3) semistructured interviews conducted at the six sites with NGOs, health officials and providers, users' committees, and members of multisectoral committees during a two-week period in December 1998.

This study will describe the context in which the Consorcio Mujer project operated, focusing on developments in the health sector in Peru. The quality of care, citizenship, and users' rights principles that guided the project's interventions will be described, and the interventions and results of the main two phases of the project will be analyzed in detail. The chapter ends with a discussion of the factors that promote and pose barriers to sustainable dialogue between community women's organizations and the health sector.

THE CONTEXT IN PERU FOR THE CONSORCIO MUJER PROJECT

Health and the Health Sector

Peru is one of the poorest countries in Latin America.[1] At the time of the Consorcio Mujer project (1993–1998), 37 percent of its 26.1 million citizens lived below the poverty line, a figure that rose to 61 percent in rural areas, according to the National Statistics Institute (1999 and 2000). The statistics on access to the health system were also bleak. According to the 1998 Human Development Report, approximately 56 percent of the population had no access to health services, and one study showed that in the period from 1995–1997, of those with health problems who did not consult a health professional, for more than 60 percent the reason was lack of financial resources.[2] There are multiple barriers to access. For example, many

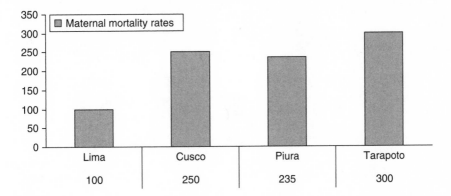

	Lima	Cusco	Piura	Tarapoto
	100	250	235	300

Figure 3.1
Regional Differences in Maternal Mortality Rates

service providers cannot easily communicate with the 27 percent of the population whose first language is Quechua, rather than Spanish.[3]

In 1997, maternal mortality was estimated at 265 maternal deaths for every 100,000 live births, one of the highest rates in Latin America.[4] The differences in health conditions and indicators between Lima and outlying departments[5] were (and continue to be) particularly marked, as Figure 3.1 shows.

The Peruvian government set an ambitious goal in early 1998 of reducing maternal mortality by 50 percent by the year 2002, but there were three important obstacles: lack of access in rural areas, failure to make childbirth services culturally appropriate, and the fees for childbirth expenses in hospitals. The last obstacle is believed to be an important factor in the low percent of women attended by health professionals in childbirth.

The level of unmet need for family planning services was also high, according to the statistics gathered in the 1996 demographic survey.[6] In rural areas, the observed fertility rate was 5.6, and the desired rate 3.1, while in urban areas, the observed rate was 2.8 and the desired rate 1.9. In 1994, one study estimated that 271,150 clandestine abortions were practiced annually in Peru, of which 47 percent presented complications.[7] Figure 3.2 on contraceptive prevalence and births attended by professionals shows the same regional disparities as for maternal mortality.[8] For this reason, the Consorcio Mujer program decided to work in three major cities outside of the capital.

Throughout the 1990s, the health sector in Peru suffered as a result of the constant reorganization in various health sector reform efforts. While the main thrust of all of these efforts was decentralization, along with a level of self-financing of the health system through users fees, in fact centralizing tendencies under Fujimori's authoritarian government[9] limited the decision-making authority of departmental health officials and their access to the income generated at the departmental level.

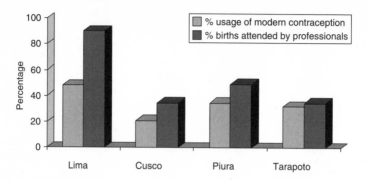

Figure 3.2
Regional Differences: Contraceptive Prevalence and Skilled Attendants at Childbirth (in %)

These tendencies of the Fujimori government undercut other democratizing initiatives in the health sector during this period. In 1992, when Consorcio Mujer conceived this project, there was little interaction between public health authorities and the women's movement. However, the time was ripe to initiate dialogue, because a new health sector reform was underway that mandated community involvement in setting priorities.[10] The reform restructured health facilities into networks of health posts reporting and referring to a secondary or tertiary-level facility. Some of these facilities were part of a pilot program: "Local Health Administration Committees" (CLAS), in which community representatives not only led needs assessments and helped set priorities, but also shared oversight of the facility with the director and other top staff. The CLAS were intended to be completely self-financed and autonomous. According to some informants, CLAS often had substantially higher user fees than the other health centers and posts.

As of December 1997 there were 548 CLAS scattered throughout the country. As is to be expected, CLAS generated mixed reactions based on both positive and negative experiences. In Lima, where the CLAS were not yet implemented at the time of this study (1999), providers spread negative rumors about community representatives representing political parties, and not users. Most relevant to this study is the ensuing atmosphere of apprehension surrounding the whole issue of community participation: the insecurity of mid-level management in Lima, which had not yet converted to the network system, and the anxiety among users about possible whole-scale increases in fees. These apprehensions mainly affected the pilot efforts in the three Lima municipalities in the Consorcio Mujer project during the years 1997 and 1998. In general, the results from this project were much more positive in the municipalities outside Lima, where decentralization and community oversight were already a fact of life.

Reproductive Rights Violations and Quality of Care in the Health System

In Peru in the late 1980s and early 1990s, both feminist organizations and established population and family planning institutions documented the nature and scope of problems with the quality of reproductive health care.[11] Feminist organizations in particular focused on widespread violations of users' rights.[12] In the early 1990s, partially influenced by USAID priorities, the Peruvian family planning program's preference for provider-dependent and long-acting methods led to an overly restrictive focus on provision of IUDs and sterilization.[13] Even though the HIV/AIDS epidemic was increasing in the country, provision of condoms was given low priority. Although significant proportions of indigenous women in Peru prefer natural methods, instead of helping women to use these methods more effectively, the public family planning program actively discouraged women from using them. After President Fujimori consolidated his hold on the government in 1992,[14] his strong focus on population control became increasingly evident, and exacerbated these tendencies.

At first, however, Fujimori's interventions seemed to favor women's rights and reproductive rights. Along with more than 180 other countries, the government of Peru signed the Programme of Action from ICPD without reservations in 1994, thus committing the Peruvian government to make individual well-being and reproductive rights—and not demographic targets—the axis of its population policy. Fujimori also gratified the Peruvian women's movement by appearing personally at the Beijing Conference (FWCW) in 1995, giving a speech that endorsed women's rights. Bucking the opposition of the Catholic Church, the Congress (controlled by the governing party) also passed legislation that relaxed the restrictions on male and female sterilization, thus expanding the range of contraceptive methods available to Peruvians.

The Peruvian government also implemented major policy and program initiatives to improve the quality of care and increase respect for human rights in the health system. In consonance with the goals of ICPD, during the 1990s, large multilateral and bilateral projects focused on improving access, infrastructure, and quality of care in reproductive health services, broadening the focus on family planning to include a major emphasis on lowering maternal mortality and on cervical cancer prevention. Some of these projects contracted women's NGOs to conduct key components designed to improve quality of care in health services.[15] Throughout the 1980s and early 1990s, these NGOs had worked closely with grassroots women community leaders in both health and community development efforts with a focus on women's empowerment. Therefore, they were very familiar with the day-to-day failures of the health services in quality of care and in meeting women's needs. Working on this issue that formed a central part of the feminist agenda vis-à-vis the health system gave the NGOs a close link with the positive goals of the Ministry of Health (MOH) in the mid-1990s.

However, beginning in 1995, Fujimori pushed highly coercive initiatives in the family planning program aimed at population control, thus working at cross-purposes with all of these positive initiatives. The NGOs' close working relationship with the MOH at this point led to sharp divisions within the women's movement regarding when, whether, and how to denounce publicly the reproductive rights abuses.[16]

Throughout the history of the Consorcio Mujer project, even as the top decision-makers in the Ministry of Health and the president's office placed a positive focus on improving quality of care, they also followed MOH's traditional *modus operandi*, which emphasized productivity and efficiency, through target-driven campaigns for vaccinations and Pap smears. When this same modus operandi was applied to demographic targets and steriliza-tion campaigns, the result was disastrous. Population control was publicly stated as a high priority for President Fujimori, who believed that it would help reduce poverty. Accordingly, from 1995–1997, the MOH implemented an intense campaign with the goal of sterilizing two million Peruvian women—supposedly the number of women in recent demographic surveys who wanted no more children and were not sterilized. According to most accounts, the president's office worked directly with the MOH to impose and keep track of progress on unofficial but inflexible monthly quotas for numbers of sterilizations at the regional level, descending to the level of each health facility and each provider within a facility. Providers and directors faced both threats and incentives to meet their individual and facility-level quotas. Given their low pay and, for many, lack of job stability,[17] few providers could afford to ignore these pressures.

This period in the history of the Peruvian health system was characterized by these contradictory trends—some of which protected and promoted rights while others led to rights abuses. During the height of the sterilization campaigns, the quality of care campaigns continued, and efforts to halt the rights abuses gained an important legal instrument when the Peruvian Congress passed the new General Health Law No. 26842 in July 1997, with a very progressive section on users' rights. The Consorcio Mujer NGOs built on this important policy advance, training both women and providers on users' rights as established by law, and disseminating widely a poster with a list of these rights.

THE CONSORCIO MUJER PROJECT—HISTORY AND FRAMEWORK

The project analyzed in this study was designed in the early 1990s by a consortium of six Peruvian feminist nongovernmental organizations (NGOs)[18]—Consorcio Mujer. Arising logically from the context of decen-tralizing health sector reform and quality of care initiatives, the several-stage project empowered local women to advocate for and collaborate in the improvement of reproductive health services in their own municipalities.

Each of the Consorcio Mujer NGOs participating in this project selected a community; in five out of the six communities, the NGO had a tradition of work with both providers and local women's organizations.[19] Three communities were in the Lima, and one each was in the Amazonian jungle (Tarapoto), the Andean highlands (Cusco), and on the rural coast (Piura)—representing the main cultural/geographic zones in Peru.

The strategy was to involve both local women community leaders and service providers, first in assessing the quality of care, and then in training on users' rights, followed by direct dialogue about how to respond to the assessments. This project required profound shifts in attitudes of both providers and community women, so that both would recognize women as self-empowered citizens with the right to high quality health care.

Each community followed a several-stage process from 1993 through 1998:[20]

Phase I: Evaluation, Feedback and Dissemination

- Participatory evaluations of quality of services in a whole health district, involving health providers, the NGO, and community women's organizations.
- Multisectoral meetings to discuss the findings, and dissemination of the findings in a publication.
- A media campaign in each community on quality of care and users' rights.

Phase II: Pilot Interventions in Quality Improvement

- Simultaneous training of providers in one key clinic in the community and women community leaders from the clinic's catchment area in quality of care and users' rights.
- Identification of quality of care issues in the clinic by both providers and users, and development of concrete proposals for improvement by each.
- Workshops on quality of care and users' rights carried out by the trained women leaders among their community organizations.
- Meetings with trained providers and users to present their proposals for service improvements to each other, and develop a consensus work plan to address the quality issues.
- Formation of quality committees among providers and users' defense committees among the users to promote ongoing dialogue on quality issues. This component was designed to be the main mechanism to sustain the impact of the project once funding ended.

Citizenship, Users' Rights, and Quality of Care

Being citizens in our dealings with the health services means that we assume that health is a social right that we hold in order to achieve well-being. We strengthen our capacity to act with autonomy, knowing our rights as users of the health services, and participating actively in decision making about our health, so that we assume responsibility for these decisions. We participate in the running of the health services, giving our opinions on the quality of care, presenting proposals and suggestions for improvement, and demanding these when necessary.[21]

Linking quality of care in health services to women's citizenship and sexual and reproductive rights was a logical and coherent step for the feminist consortium. As Latin American countries underwent democratization in the 1980s and 1990s, the concept of citizenship emerged within the Latin American women's movement as the theoretical and political foundation of discussions about women's status and empowerment. In order for women to exercise full citizenship, both the society at large and individual women would need to recognize female rights and autonomy in all spheres of life (for example, occupational, political, economic, cultural, religious, and sexual). Women who enjoy full citizenship have the power, confidence, and appropriate channels for political participation in order to defend their rights in these spheres. A truly democratic society would thereby imply a shift from female dependence and submission toward equality and power sharing in governance and in the myriad decisions that affect women's lives.[22]

The citizenship model stands in contrast to the paternalistic model, which is based on the belief that services for the poor are a matter of charity, not of the human right to health. A corollary is that the provider knows what is best for the user. Sensitive to past and current abuses, the consortium emphasized users' rights related to voluntary use of health care services, informed consent, nondiscrimination, and access to high-quality health care, regardless of ethnic group or socioeconomic class. Table 3.1 provides a comparison of the citizenship and paternalistic models of health care.

Table 3.1
Comparison of Two Models of Health Care Provision

Citizenship Model	Paternalistic Model
Users have rights of access to high-quality health services, to freedom of choice, and to be treated with dignity.	Health services benefit users, and are provided to low-income people as a favor or charity.
Community participation means that users are involved in setting goals.	Community participation means that community organizations help achieve providers' goals.
Horizontal relationships: Providers listen to users' concerns nonjudgmentally, and their responses consider these concerns.	Hierarchical relationships: Providers know what is best for the users, or "patients."

In applying this concept of citizenship to the health sector, Consorcio Mujer emphasized community participation and users' rights. To Consorcio Mujer, community participation meant that users should participate in setting goals for health care provision and in helping providers achieve these goals. Communities organizing for access to health care are more effective when they believe that they are fighting for entitlements rather than requesting charity. When providers believe that they are providing services as a favor, they react angrily when users complain about the quality of services, but when providers believe that these services are the right of all citizens, they are more apt to perceive quality complaints as legitimate. One quote from a health center director in Lima illustrates the paradigm shift that the Consorcio program aimed for. "Before the providers were the authority, and the patients asked us to help them as a favor. Now we say, 'We are employed thanks to the patients.' "[23]

To appeal to goals that were already paramount in the health sector's agenda, Consorcio Mujer framed its project as one that would improve quality of health care. To unite the concepts of quality and citizenship, the consortium placed users' rights and women's participation at the center of the concept of quality, building on the quality of care framework developed by Judith Bruce for family planning programs. This framework recommends ample choices of methods, complete and appropriate information, respectful and high-quality provider-client interaction, technical competence, continuity of care, and access to a range of related services.[24] The users' rights framework used by Consorcio Mujer added the following principles:[25]

- Respect for users' rights is central to the concept of quality. User satisfaction is important but not sufficient. When women don't view themselves as subjects of rights, they blame themselves when they are mistreated, and don't express dissatisfaction with services.

- Major emphasis is placed on informed consent, freedom of choice and voluntarism, and respect for dignity of the person. The Consorcio's training highlighted the concept of freedom of choice to counteract coercive pressures on both providers and users in sterilization campaigns.

- Users have the right to privacy and confidentiality. Peruvian women complained about the presence of third parties without their consent, and about frequent intrusions into examining rooms.

- The right of users to express opinions and organize is a progressive feature of Peruvian General Health Law #26842, passed in 1997, and was a key axis of the Consorcio Mujer program.

- Nondiscrimination based on sex, religion, race, civil status, or location is enshrined in the Health Law. Consorcio Mujer added in their list of users' rights: nondiscrimination on the basis of economic status, age, and sexual orientation. (Discrimination on the basis of economic status was a frequent quality complaint in the six sites of the Consorcio Mujer program.)

- The right to culturally appropriate treatment and services is key for ethnic minorities. The Consorcio Mujer organizations believe that lack of attention to this right is an important factor in the underuse of maternity hospitals in Peru.
- The right of access to the widest range of services entails addressing barriers of geographical distance and cost. Cost became a major issue in Peru with the increasing users' fees.

Addressing these issues, Consorcio Mujer focused on the empowerment of users in three ways:

1. teaching women self-care, so that they are less dependent on the medical establishment for maintaining health;
2. educating them on gender and human rights issues to increase their view of themselves as bearers of rights; and
3. providing strategies to defend their rights as users of health services and as citizens.

PHASE ONE: PARTICIPATORY ASSESSMENTS OF QUALITY OF CARE

In 1994, Consorcio Mujer began gathering information within the six communities on how both users and providers viewed quality of care. A number of studies had documented these issues in the past, but had concentrated on family planning; only two had incorporated clients' perspectives. Therefore, the consortium's evaluations included a dual focus on women's own perceptions of health care, and on the health services' quality, including the capacity to provide a full range of women's health services. The evaluation examined capacity for and the quality of basic gynecologic, contraceptive, and obstetric services, including the diagnosis and treatment of reproductive tract infections.

In the six municipalities, the appointed NGO used standardized instruments to survey providers and at least thirty users, and to conduct direct observations of provider-client interactions, with the clients' permission, in small health posts, larger health centers, and maternity hospitals. Some questions were specific, but many were open-ended, for example, "Was there any point during the medical visit when you felt ashamed?"[26]

The findings documented a range of problems:[27]

- *Disrespectful treatment.* Women reported being subjected to insults, angry shouting, and belittling. Nearly half (48 percent) suggested the need for improvement in providers' interpersonal skills. When asked which aspects of health care were most important for building trust, 57 percent highlighted "good treatment." In all, 17–30 percent of respondents in each municipality felt shame because of being rebuked or belittled by a provider. One user from the highlands testified: "I don't go to the hospital because women are treated terribly, when they cry or scream with pain, the nurses ... insult them, 'Is this how you screamed when you were conceiving?' ... so I feel fear and shame."

- *Providers' failure to greet users and introduce themselves.* The proportion of providers who greeted the client ranged from 15 to 60 percent. The project gave high importance to this indicator, which enables accountability. Women need to know the name of a provider who has mistreated them in order to lodge complaints.

- *Waiting time.* Waiting time was more than one hour for 48 percent of women. However, women tended to be resigned to the waiting time, but were outraged when they perceived that the "first-come, first-served" rule was violated.

- *Inadequate information.* Women complained of perfunctory and incomplete counseling. For example, they reported that providers did not explain diagnostic procedures and follow-up treatment. Many felt the explanations offered were not fully understandable. Only 17 percent of providers gave any explanations before or during vaginal exams, for example. In Cusco and Piura, only 8 to 9 percent of providers explained Pap smears, and only 9 to 23 percent provided information on breast self-exams. According to Consorcio Mujer staff, "The information given to users is scant. ... When users have vaginal infections, generally the professional says, 'It's inflamed'."[28]

- *Interruptions, lack of privacy, and presence of third parties.* Women described frequent interruptions by other personnel while they were undergoing exams. Because of the presence of third parties (mostly medical students), 28 percent had no privacy during their exam; 8 to 19 percent felt shame because of this. Overall, 60 percent of women reported feeling shame at exposing their genitals. (Although one might expect that such modesty would lead to preference for a female provider, only 10 percent of respondents rated having a female provider as being of high importance.)

The findings were compiled into a report and discussed with local women's organizations, frontline providers, and municipal health authorities. These discussions often took place under the auspices of multisectoral committees—organized by the government in the mid-1990s to provide regular opportunities for communication between private and public actors involved in promoting health in a region or district.[29] The discussions were designed to reach agreement about courses of action to remedy the problems identified. There were difficulties, however, in attaining an adequate response from local authorities. Although the local women's groups and the frontline providers were dedicated to the process, they were not in a position to effect changes throughout large municipalities. The providers and users who had participated in the evaluation were from several health centers in the region, hence the findings could not be applied directly to improve services at any one center. Furthermore, because the decentralization of the health sector was still in its initial stages, central-level guidelines were still defining many municipal work plans.

The experience in Piura, the only rural area included in the consortium's project, exemplifies the challenges of having an impact on service delivery through this strategy. A daylong assembly was convened to review the outcomes of the quality of care evaluation.[30] Centro IDEAS, the NGO consortium member that had conducted the evaluation, other NGOs, the Rural Women's Network,[31] all of the midwives in the area, and municipal authorities attended.

Midwives presented findings from the provider interviews, and women from the community presented a summary of users' focus groups. In addition to deficiencies in service quality, women had highlighted the need to address neglected health problems such as domestic violence. Comments from both midwives and women from the community noted the need for more comprehensive services. However, when the midwives presented their work-plan for the year, it was as if these reports had never been made. The central authorities had already mandated two campaigns promoting and providing free Pap smears and free sterilization. An NGO representative stood up and asked, "Wait a minute. What does this have to do with everything we just heard?" However, there was no possibility of adjustment; funding was tied to directives from Lima.

While the municipal discussions led to frustration, the interaction between women and providers was generally viewed as valuable. For example, in the Piura meeting, users complained that while the Pap smears provided through the campaigns were free, when women returned for their results, they were often told to pay a fee for the clinic visit. Not surprisingly, some women from this poverty-stricken rural region went home without their results. These complaints helped providers grasp the frustration and distrust such campaigns generated in the community.

In addition to facilitating discussion, Consorcio Mujer used two other tactics to promote users' rights as the linchpin of quality of care. First, it designed a public media campaign with the slogan "Let's Be Citizens, Not Patients!" and distributed literature as part of the country's Safe Motherhood Day campaign. Second, the consortium redoubled its efforts to influence the quality-of-care evaluations at the central levels of the Ministry of Health, and offered the ministry use of its research instruments and outcome indicators. These negotiations, initially promising, were truncated as controversy over the government's sterilization campaigns led to a growing rift between the ministry and some of the NGOs in the consortium.

At a joint meeting, the Consorcio Mujer members reflected on the experiences in Phase One, and concluded that while the assessments and dissemination had served to raise consciousness about common quality of health care problems, more targeted interventions would be necessary to produce actual changes at the clinic level. They designed Phase Two of the project so that concrete improvements in quality of care at key clinics could serve a demonstration effect within each department.

PHASE TWO: COMMUNITY PARTICIPATION IN QUALITY IMPROVEMENT

The new strategy focused on: (1) collecting site-specific data regarding quality and capacity of participating health centers; (2) using the data in training courses with both clients and providers; (3) generating consensus on specific recommendations for improvements; and (4) creating sustainable mechanisms for dialogue between health providers and users.

As a first step in the new strategy, the participating NGOs met with municipal health officials to select one health center in each project area. With an eye toward replicating the project beyond these pilot sites, the NGOs chose health centers that had been designated "network coordinators" as part of the national decentralization scheme in health sector reform programs.[32]

Quality Assessments in Each Clinic

As mentioned above, while the results of the 1994 user surveys were useful for diagnosing general quality of care problems in the health services in a geographic region, the sampling strategy did not provide any one center with a reliable assessment of quality of care. In 1997, Consorcio Mujer conducted new provider and user surveys on quality of care at each of the six pilot centers. The most common user complaints paralleled the findings of the 1994 evaluation: disrespectful treatment, long waiting time, lack of privacy, and inadequate information. A number of new complaints surfaced in the 1997 surveys,[33] however, including:

- *Pressure to be sterilized or accept intrauterine devices.* Overt and systematic pressure on providers to persuade users to be sterilized had not yet emerged at the time of the 1994 evaluation, but was evident in the 1997 surveys.[34] As a community health promoter in Carabayllo, Lima, reported in 1998, "Last year they made the mama tie her tubes, whether she wanted to or not, like a kid who has to obey the father's rules."[35]

- *Lack of culturally appropriate services.* Failure to respect Quechua childbirth practices was of concern in all six sites.[36] The incompatibility between modern hospital-based childbirth practices and Andean customs (see Box 3.1) has long been common knowledge in Peru and is one of the main obstacles to increasing rates of hospital-based births.

- *Mistreatment and fee collection.* Ironically, the health sector reform's focus on achieving financial autonomy for local health services—potentially a significant barrier to access for low-income Peruvians—increased attention to quality of care in the public health centers and posts. However, certain perverse incentives in the policies also undermined quality of care. The collection of fees is a relatively new practice in the public sector, and the money collected is retained by health centers to purchase supplies and equipment, but most importantly to supplement the low salaries of permanent employees.[37] As a result, users at five sites reported problems with

Box 3.1
Traditional Andean vs. Modern Medical Birthing Practices

> Andean women traditionally labor in a warm and dark environment among family members and/or traditional midwives. They ingest certain hot broths and teas, and the customary position when giving birth is to squat with the use of a birth pole. Postpartum practices include a restricted diet and burial of the placenta. The Western hospital model, with cool light rooms, enforcement of a prone position, and automatic disposal of the placenta, is particularly uncongenial to these women, and helps explain the low percentage of women whose births are attended by professionals. Indigenous women are often subjected to racist comments and mistreatment as well.[38]

providers charging for services that are officially free of charge. Furthermore, women at all six sites reported mistreatment of indigent women who requested fee waivers. Because every request for a fee waiver potentially reduced the salary of the person considering the request, it is small wonder that the requests generated ill will! A users' committee member in Cusco explained, "If we have money, they treat us well. ... [Rural women] don't like to come to the city to give birth, because they have no money; the doctor ignores them and the nurses yell at them and insult them."

The survey asked users to characterize good-quality treatment as well, and many willingly discussed positive experiences in the health system, again emphasizing the importance of personal interaction:[39]

She treats me kindly. I have a lot of trust and confidence in her and she is a good doctor. Several friends and I see her and we like her a lot.
She calls me by my name, and doesn't say anything negative about my having sexual relations and not being married; in other places they scold you.
She talks to me like a sister so that I'm not afraid during my labor; she helps me get off the bed and gives me advice.

The Training Workshops

Consorcio Mujer developed separate but parallel workshops on quality of care, users' rights, and sexual and reproductive rights for providers from the pilot health center and women leaders from its catchment area. Direct service providers, auxiliary nursing staff, and, in some settings, the health center director attended the providers' workshops. For the users' workshop, the consortium NGOs invited leaders of community-based organizations (such as food committees and mothers' clubs) who also worked as health promoters.[40] Consorcio Mujer selected these women because they had enough health and leadership experience to replicate the workshop in the community. Most of these women were poor and had only primary-level education.

Each workshop consisted of four half-day sessions. The goals for participants were to:

- understand the concepts of sexual and reproductive rights and users' rights, including the content in the new health law;[41]
- critically analyze the attitudes and assumptions underlying the paternalistic model of health care;
- reflect on their own experiences as users of health services, paying particular attention to problems identified in the surveys;
- generate new models of provider-client interaction through practical exercises in new ways of communicating and relating to each other;
- generate concrete proposals for improving quality at each health center.

Consorcio Mujer trainers used various communication strategies to promote reflection about quality-of-care issues and to stimulate positive role-playing. For example, participants analyzed an actual provider-client transaction that was recorded during the 1994 evaluations (see Box 3.2). These participatory and intensive techniques built skills and enabled attitude change.[42]

The consortium training emphasized different issues in the providers' and users' workshops. Providers dealt first with their own experiences as users and with users' rights, and then concentrated on issues related to quality. Providers also discussed the tension between quality and productivity, and quality-improvement strategies. Users dealt with self-esteem, rights, citizenship, and gender issues before they turned to the topic of quality of care. The women leaders were also trained to conduct workshops on these issues for their community organizations, an outcome that was not expected of the providers.

Box 3.3 illustrates two training exercises, one for providers and one for users, which addressed central issues for each group.

In the final stage of the training, participants in both workshops developed specific proposals for improving services and formed implementation teams. After the training, the Consorcio NGOs coordinated a joint meeting between the two groups to develop a consensus plan for quality improvement. The expected result from the meeting was that the providers would form quality committees to implement these proposals, while the community leaders would form users' defense committees to promote their suggestions, with the two groups engaging in ongoing dialogue.

Box 3.2
Speaking to Deaf Ears: An Exercise to Analyze a Provider-Client Interaction[43]

The user is aged twenty-four, a high school graduate and a market vendor. She has come to the clinic because of a delayed menstrual period and received a positive pregnancy test result. The provider is a midwife with twenty years of experience.

Provider: Sit down, my love. [She asks the number of children (2) and the date of last period.] Little mother (*madrecita*), did you do a Pregnostic (pregnancy test)?
User: Yes, doctor. (She gives her the lab report.)
Provider: Who prescribed this?
User: I did. I came to the Center and took the test, but I don't want to have more children now, I have many problems.
Provider: What's going on here, little girl (*niñita*)?* Why don't you want to be pregnant?
User: (Laughs very nervously) Things are not well at home, we are still building the house, and I have no money.
Provider: Do you have sons or daughters?
User: Two daughters
Provider: So many little women? Now let's try for the little man. We're going to have this little child, the last one, *madrecita*, because then we'll take care of you with pills or little tubes in your arm. Look, like these [shows the pictures of oral contraceptives and Norplant]. We won't do anything foolish, we'll respect this little boy child, and we'll love him very much as well.
User: I was taking Lo Femenal, so why did I get pregnant?
Provider: You didn't take them correctly, my daughter (*mi hijita*).
User: No. I took them correctly.
Provider: But surely, you forgot one.
User: No, I didn't.
Provider: I'm going to give you some pills so that you don't get nauseous. Next time you come, I'll do your analyses.
User: But Doctor, I'm not nauseous.
Provider: It doesn't matter, take them anyway, they'll be good for you. [She doesn't indicate how many times a day, or for how long.]

*Peruvian feminist NGOs have insisted that eliminating the common use of diminutive names such as found in this interview is an important element in the empowerment of the female user and in constructing more horizontal relationships. When challenged on this practice, providers typically respond that these labels are a sign of warmth and affection, and an important part of putting the client at ease. However, these labels clearly signal a vertical relationship; no one can imagine an indigenous woman calling a nurse "*niñita*."

Response to the Workshops[44]

Reactions Among Providers

The providers were committed to participating in the workshop. In many sites, the sessions lasted for several hours beyond the scheduled

Box 3.3
Sample Exercises from Providers' and Users' Training

Users Training Module: "YOUR DAY IN COURT"

Objective: To enable women to defend principles of reproductive rights in the face of arguments to the contrary.

1. Group discussion on the list of reproductive rights. The group chooses the right to choose what they think is most important to work on.

2. Three women become the jury, and the rest of the group divides into defenders of the rights and opponents. In the opponents' group, each woman is assigned a role with a card worn on the chest, such as bishop, neighbor, husband, *machista* [sexist man], scientist, chief doctor, etc. The defenders' group represents the community women.

3. After each group organizes its arguments, people from each group alternate by speaking for one minute.

4. At the end, the jury decides whether the right is approved or not.

Providers Training Module—Paper Boat Exercise

Objective: To encourage providers to examine the trade-off between quality goals and productivity.

1. The facilitator shows the group how to make a well-made paper boat, and gives each small group thirty sheets, with the instructions that they have three minutes to make twenty boats. The group that makes the most well-made boats wins the prize. Points are subtracted for torn or misshapen sheets.

2. In the next stage, the facilitator delivers thirty sheets to each group, with the instructions to make thirty boats in three minutes.

3. The judges compare the quality of the boats produced between the first and second stages. (Invariably, the second stage sees more quality problems.)

4. The group discusses the relevance of the exercise to their discussions on quality of care, and the productivity goals set by the ministry.

5. The group discusses the use of productivity goals to evaluate professionals or services. Messages reinforced by facilitator at this stage: improving quality may lower productivity in the short-term, but in the long-term, it results in less "waste," as in the discarded boats. Quality attracts more users to the center, and costs less when the problems of the users are adequately dealt with in one visit.

time, sometimes until 10:30 P.M. In one site, an unsympathetic administrator scheduled an obligatory meeting to conflict with the workshop; the staff reacted by rescheduling the session for the evening, after work hours.

In general, providers demonstrated openness to learning, recognized the need for quality improvement, and were aware of remaining obstacles, including a need for further training to deal with gender and sexuality issues.

Providers' comments point to adjustments in their own attitudes, as well as to a realistic appraisal of the long-term nature of the change process demanded of them:

We have to be realistic. We have been raised a certain way and consciously we know how we should be, but we can't live up to it. We have realized the problem that it is difficult to work on these issues with the community when we ourselves still have machismo inside us.

We learned that the users wanted us to ask them about sexuality. So now, we ask in a friendly way. But we still have some prejudices, and have asked Centro IDEAS for more training.

The focus on the "internal client" in the workshop seemed to be a powerful tool for change. One clinic director remarked:

They gave information on users' rights to us and to the users, thus initiating communication between us. Before this, we had problems, because we saw things one way, and they saw them in another. The exercise where we put ourselves in the shoes of the users—[in which I was] remembering a time when I was treated terribly—influenced me. No one paid attention to me, and I got very demoralized.

In all six sites, the discussions on the tension between productivity and quality revealed providers' frustrations at feeling pulled between a concern for users' rights and institutional pressures to sterilize women. As one doctor in a Piura training session exclaimed, "What about my rights? Who is going to look out for me when I apply quality principles and am fired for not meeting my quotas?"[45]

In analyzing quality problems in provider-client interactions, the providers also pointed to the anger and frustration that they feel when—in their opinion—users do not fulfill their obligations. One provider from Piura echoed sentiments expressed in most of the other sites as well: "And when the women know their rights, what about their responsibilities? For example, when they don't follow our instructions for treatment, or don't respect the clinic's schedule."

Reactions Among Users

The response among users was equally favorable. The training used participatory methods to support each participant's ability to "reconstruct oneself as a bearer of rights." Before the Consorcio project, the training provided by Peruvian NGOs with these grassroots women's organizations had focused on improving their effectiveness as community leaders, that is, on what the women could do for others. Consorcio Mujer NGOs viewed the linkage of personal issues in women's lives (for example lack of self-esteem and recurrent RTIs) with their ability to organize with others for their rights as citizens as particularly effective.[46]

A trainer in Piura summed up this process:

What is new about the module is the concept of citizenship and rights. While the women already had some idea of these concepts, they were able to internalize them. The women reflected deeply. At the beginning of the training, they said that the quality of the services was just fine. Then, as we probed more into the different aspects of users' rights, the incidents of violations emerged—having to do with lack of privacy, inadequate information, mistreatment....

At the beginning, I didn't think that the women were going to open up, but I was wrong. Little by little, they began to talk about everything they had left unsaid, and to express it with all their emotions. One woman wept as she described how she had been humiliated. The providers understood users' rights much more easily than the users did.... [For the users] it was difficult to grasp the concept, because they only envisioned themselves as users and not as bearers of rights.

This experience points out the limitations of traditional user satisfaction surveys. Women who do not view themselves as bearers of rights often do not express dissatisfaction. The user trainees in Consorcio Mujer's project voiced pride in their increased ability to ask questions, complain about mistreatment, resist coercion, and engage in discussion with providers on quality issues.

We didn't know about self-esteem. We learned to love and value our bodies and ourselves. Before, we let ourselves be mistreated, but no longer.

The concept of users' rights was new; it fit us like a ring on a finger.... We had complained before but without legal grounds.

Now we understand that human rights include the right to health. This caused us to think deeply. Why do we let them mistreat us? Why aren't we capable of reacting or asking for what we want?

The emphasis on self-esteem was important. We learned we can say no. We give and give, always for others.... Women always feel guilty.

I had decided not to get my tubes tied, but then one day a very angry nurse came to my house and asked, "Why would you want more children if you can't feed them?" I replied, "Miss, I'm not going to do it and no one can make me." Because if I want to, they can tie them, and if I don't, they can't force me. The nurse came for the second time, but I didn't want to meet her.... I had already been trained, so I told her that no one could make me, that this is my right and my body.

The Experience of Replicating the Training

After the training, the community health promoters replicated the training in users' rights among the members of their organizations. In all six sites, this was a new and empowering experience for these community leaders, and expanded the impact of the training. The manual developed by the NGO for the user training had to be adapted and simplified greatly for this purpose since many members of the community organizations have little or incomplete primary education. Even for the most experienced health promoters involved, this was their first experience in serving as trainers, that is, taking over the traditional role of the more professional NGOs.

All the promoters interviewed commented on how nervous it made them to assume this new role with their constituencies, on the one hand, but on the other hand, they revealed what an opportunity it posed for their own growth and leadership development. The leaders of the Salitral [Piura] network commented: "One just has to get over feeling nervous and learn to be strong, and capable of communicating new ideas to our groups....We divided the work [for the training in each community] and each of us gave at least one of the sessions. [Q: And how did the workshops go?] Some women were very ashamed and timid, but as the sessions progressed they relaxed."

Consorcio Mujer hurried to implement this phase of the program because they felt such urgency about disseminating the message on users' rights effectively, to a broader audience, as the government's sterilization campaigns continued. Even though the campaigns officially ended in early 1998, it took some time for them to wind down and for NGOs and community organizations to verify this. Furthermore, the campaigns left a legacy of fear and distrust. Therefore, it was still urgent to convince community women that they were strong enough to defend their rights and to inform them of strategies that they could use in case of mistreatment or attempted coercion. The Consorcio hoped that given these tools, women would not deprive themselves of needed care at the health centers out of feelings of fear and distrust.

AGREEING ON SOLUTIONS

The results suggest that the Consorcio's intervention among providers and users was highly effective in producing concrete changes in the participating centers. In four of the six sites, providers formed quality committees and users formed user defense committees that were still functioning three to four months after their training ended. In five of the six sites,[47] the providers responded to the intervention process by instituting improvements recommended during the training workshops. However, only in the three sites outside of Lima were the changes implemented because of jointly agreed-on plans. The Lima sites only implemented ideas that arose in the provider training sessions. Several NGO trainers suggested that this difference is mainly due to the greater progress in devolving authority to departmental health officials outside of Lima; the Lima-based services tended to be still mainly under central MOH authority at the time of the study interviews in late 1998. Table 3.2 summarizes the dialogue results at each site.

In the sites where the joint dialogue process was implemented as planned, the focus of post-training meetings was on reaching agreements to solve the quality of care problems identified in the health center. Each group came to these meetings equipped with a new perspective about the rights of users and with concrete suggestions to solve quality of care problems, developed in the final sessions of the training. In these follow-up meetings, the two committees communicated their suggestions to each other, and they reached agreement on a joint list of remedies, with a work plan to implement them in which quality and users committees shared responsibilities.

Although only limited evaluations of quality have been carried out since these measures were instituted, providers and users in all six sites interviewed in 1998 testified that services, while not perfect, have improved. Follow-up training of providers has consolidated some gains, while staff turnover has eroded others. Providers' comments pointed to serious commitment to quality improvement, and to remaining areas of concern:

We made the changes needed and applied a second survey, and we saw improvements in satisfaction with admissions, the cashier, and the first aid room. However, our basic problem is that we have few personnel and many patients. The problem of waiting time cannot be solved.

The following list includes solutions implemented at one or more of the sites.

Promoting respectful treatment

- Rotate staff who treat users well into positions requiring public contact. In one Lima site, for example, a friendly cleaning woman was promoted to admissions.
- Establish procedures for firing, transferring, or disciplining personnel who are consistently the focus of mistreatment complaints. A doctor in the same Lima site lost her post as clinic director because of community pressure.
- Provide follow-up training to address assumptions and attitudes underlying rude behavior.

Ensuring that providers introduce themselves

- Require providers to wear name badges.

Reducing waiting time

- Create chart retrieval routines to limit waiting time for women who arrive without their health cards.

- Post someone to direct clients to their proper destination.
- Systematically enforce procedures to serve clients in the order in which they arrive.

Protecting privacy

- Establish a private area in which a user can state the reason for her visit.
- Place signs on examination room doors indicating whether the room is "free" or "occupied."

Countering pressures from the sterilization campaigns

- Establish a waiting period between the counseling visit and the sterilization procedure. (This practice, originally instituted in one site, has now become part of the Ministry of Health's guidelines.)
- Conduct a community survey to prove to officials that there is no unmet need for sterilization to decrease pressure to fulfill unrealistic quotas.

Counseling

- Enforce a fifteen-minute minimum consulting time to compel providers to spend more time offering information and counseling.

Promoting cultural sensitivity

- Introduce selected elements of natural childbirth and allow women to give birth in the squatting position with family members present.
- Use Quechua-speaking auxiliary staff to translate for users during visits.

Ensuring access and appropriate fee-collection practices

- Enforce guidelines on free services.
- Establish a savings plan during antenatal visits to cover childbirth expenses (obstetric care is free but supplies must be paid for by the patient).

BARRIERS AND FACILITATING FACTORS TO DIALOGUE AND JOINT ACTIONS

Barriers to Dialogue and Partnership

Throughout the project, the relationship between health providers and community health promoters was fraught with tensions in five of the six sites in the project.[48] In the paternalistic model of "community participation" in these communities, health promoters volunteer their time to coordinate with health centers and posts to help achieve goals set by the health sector. This lack of participation in setting goals combined with the MOH's strong focus on productivity and meeting targets, resulting in providers treating health promoters as mere agents to help them increase coverage. In return, the promoters were given no compensation, even for travel costs, no official recognition, and often, no respect. As one promoter from Lima stated: "When they cannot meet their goals for coverage, they call us." Many community health promoters fiercely resented continuing to receive peremptory commands from health care providers as the predominant style of interaction: "Bring us 30 women on Tuesday for Pap smears." Without a process of horizontal dialogue, community women were unable to sympathize with the often-untenable position of the poorly paid and overstressed health professionals, who were threatened with dismissal if they did not meet their targets. The Consorcio project was designed to promote just such dialogue, but in some cases, the tensions were not fully aired.

Difficulties also arose from providers' resistance to users' new status and sense of entitlement. In one site, providers did not appreciate having users' comments included in the performance evaluations of individual care providers. In another site, the users' committee tried wearing special aprons to signify a semiofficial status, and they joined the staff when they opened the waiting room suggestion boxes and reviewed users' comments. Although this action was negotiated by Consorcio Mujer and both sides agreed in principle, it did not work in practice. A committee member explained, "One woman went to the meeting to discuss the complaints, but she found that the language they used was too sophisticated. The women from the Mothers' Club didn't want to go any more, and the providers felt invaded."

Another factor posing an obstacle to progress was the division and lack of autonomy of many community-based women's organizations during the mid-to-late 1990s in Peru. In many communities in the 1980s and early 1990s, sharp divisions arose as the Shining Path and MRTA guerrillas infiltrated community organizations. Because the terrorists targeted community leaders for assassination, many community organizations—including the women's groups—weakened greatly during this period as their original leadership resigned or went into hiding, while Shining Path designated leaders who would support them. Once the threat of Shining Path diminished in 1993–1994, the patronage of the Fujimori government took over, and the women's organizations became dependent on the municipalities, which too often meant being dependent on the political party in control. As a result, there were parallel sets of community leaders in the ubiquitous "Cup of Milk" Program and among Mother's Clubs in some communities where the Consorcio Mujer project worked. The lack of a unified community women's leadership at the municipal or subregional level made dialogue difficult.

In most sites, the NGOs had a long history of work with both the health center and the local women leaders and could build on previously established trust to facilitate the process of dialogue. The exception proves the rule. In Carabayllo, the Consorcio Mujer NGO CESIP was reaching out to a completely new geographical area, one in which the local women's organizations had had a confrontational relationship with the health system. CESIP lacked sufficient history with these organizations to influence their stance and enable an effective dialogue. According to the providers, members of the users' defense committee arrived unannounced and sat in the waiting room observing. When asked what they wanted, the women said, "We're here to supervise you." These providers refused to negotiate directly with the users' defense committee, explaining, "This community is very combative. We were afraid to enter into a formal relationship with them because we don't have the means to live up to their expectations."

Factors in Successful and Sustainable Dialogue

In spite of these barriers to establishing a more horizontal working relationship, in five of the six sites the relationship between community leaders and providers remained friendly and cooperative after the workshops. An NGO trainer in one site observed, "We have not noticed a negative reaction from the providers to women's participation. They view the women as allies."

This study's findings suggest that the post-training dialogues were most effective when the NGO had carefully negotiated and clarified the terms of the dialogue and prepared both groups in advance. In Cusco, the NGO and the Health Center agreed on how users would evaluate quality, and the promoters were well-received. The NGO also facilitated attitude change among the community leaders so that they could enter into this new kind of relationship. One leader from Cusco remarked: "We had a positive attitude...that we were there to help them reach the people most in need. Before, we just criticized and didn't offer to help." Box 3.4 illustrates the potential for quality improvement when both providers and community members negotiate in this positive spirit.

The Role of Multisectoral Committees

In theory, the existence of functioning multisectoral committees should have been a key factor in facilitating dialogue between these community-based leaders and the health providers. In fact, Table 3.2 suggests that this is not the case, and the interviews brought out the reason: barriers to including community-based grassroots leaders in committees made up mostly of professionals—whether from NGOs or government agencies. Only in Tarapoto were community organizations routinely involved in the committee meetings. The results from Tarapoto make it clear that when such

Box 3.4
Negotiating Solutions in Piura—Male Involvement

In the users' workshop, the women connected their most-mentioned health problems to their "triple role" as spouses, mothers, and workers: vaginal infections, urinary tract infections, and headaches. Discussions about the vaginal infections led the participants to recognize the urgent need for the health center to do more to reach out to their spouses.... The providers were also concerned that almost 90 percent of the women attending the center had vaginal infections and their spouses refused to be treated, and so the problem was never resolved. Accordingly, both the women and providers proposed close coordination to plan outreach to the men in their communities.

Mentioned in the workshop document as causes of the problem were: "machismo and low self-esteem of men, because when they come to the Center, it is seen as a sign of weakness" and "lack of dissemination about the services offered to the men." The women explained the problem: "For the husbands, it is shameful to go to the Health Center with their wives. Their friends will tease them, saying, 'I see that she's ordering you around.'" By December 1998, the Center had organized three workshops for men on RTIs and STIs in three different villages and was about to hold a fourth, coordinating closely with the women so that the times would be convenient and the workshops would be publicized among the neighbors. The men of Salitral asked for another workshop. All locations indicated that the best time for workshops for men were the evenings or weekends.

Other plans and suggestions included: invitation for the spouse to be included in standard protocols for prenatal care and for STD/RTI treatment; and to take advantage of holidays and events planned by others such as Fathers' Day events, and sports events. The Quality Committee had already implemented the protocol suggestion at the time of this study.

The topic of male involvement arose again in another problem given priority: the providers' lack of acceptance of "traditional" (that is, culturally specific to this region) norms and health remedies. Specifically, the women asked that their spouses be present during childbirth and that herbal remedies be recognized and incorporated into the treatment regimes.

participation is successful, these committees can indeed facilitate dialogue between the community and the health sector.

In most functioning committees in this study, the health sector convened the meetings, with commitments from NGOs and other members to sustain the basic costs of coordination. In Salitral/Piura, rural women couldn't get to meetings in the provincial seat, partly because there were no funds for their travel. In San Juan de Lurigancho, the community health leaders didn't see the potential importance of attending meetings and assumed a more traditional role of cooperation with initiatives decided by the committee. The NGO members believed that the community women find their meetings "boring."

Table 3.2
Factors in the Long-Term Outcome of Dialogue Between Health Centers and Community Women

	Attitudes of Health Sector Leadership	Quality of Care Outcomes in Health Center	User and Quality Committees, and State of Dialogue	Representation of Community Groups on Multisectoral Committees
Cusco	Resistant at higher levels.	Changes implemented according to jointly negotiated plan.	User & Quality Committees established. Good informal coordination at Health Center level only.	Multisectoral committee disbanded; Committee on Violence sometimes includes community.
Piura	Very favorable.	Many changes in joint proposal implemented, and joint initiatives to reach out to men.	Unstable joint quality committee, with representatives from Health Center and women's network.	Well-functioning Reproductive Health Committee and others. Rural women don't attend.
Tarapoto	Very favorable.	Major improvements due to Consorcio and Project 2000.	Quality Committee and User's Defense Committees established.	Well-functioning committee with focus on women's issues. User's Defense Committee takes part.

Site				
LIMA: Carabayllo	High turnover in Health Center Directors. Distrust of community groups.	Improvements as result of provider training only.	Separate user & provider committees; history of antagonism and no dialogue.	No committee exists.
LIMA: San Juan de Lurigancho	Favorable attitudes at subregional level.	Improvements from provider training eroded by staff turnover.*	Promoters affiliated with NGO service. No stable User Defense Committee. Pilot provider training carried out before Consorcio project, with no Quality Committee as a result.	Well-functioning Health Committee. Community leaders don't attend meetings, but participate in actions planned by the committee.
LIMA: San Juan de Miraflores	Sub-regional officials antagonistic to project.	Improvements as result of provider training.	Informal but cordial dialogue at Health Center level. Promoters' group affiliated with NGO service. No stable Users' Committee.	Health Center Director taking first steps to convene the community to set priorities, as part of the health sector reform process.

*Much more time had elapsed between the initial training and the author's interviews in this site than in the other five sites. Centro Flora Tristan conducted the training at the Maternity Clinic in 1995–1996, while all of the other sites conducted the training in 1998.

These experiences suggest that multisectoral committees need to involve community-based organizations meaningfully in their deliberations in order to serve as a facilitating factor for partnerships and dialogue between the health sector and the community. Involving the professional staff of NGOs alone is not enough.

The evidence from this study suggests that the following factors might promote the sustainability of continuing dialogue between community organizations and the health sector:[49]

- *Support among high-level officials for community participation as part of health sector reform.* The new health sector reform in Peru was much more advanced in the provinces than it was in Lima. Peru's reform included a process of involving the community in setting health sector priorities and a transformation of health centers into self-sufficient entities with community oversight boards. In the provinces, the hard work of convincing providers of the benefits of community oversight was well underway, while the main attitude in Lima municipalities was one of anxiety and fear, fueled by rumors of instances where the process had gone badly elsewhere. To the extent that a "culture" of community participation deepens in Peru, the committees set up under this project—or some variation of them—would tend to continue into the future.

- *The presence of other large programs working on quality of care, including pilot health sector reform.* The World Bank, USAID, and UNFPA were all strongly pushing quality of care initiatives during the project period. In one case, in Tarapoto, the Consorcio Mujer training laid the foundation for a much more ambitious quality improvement initiative called Project 2000. As one provider said, "After the training, Project 2000 fit us like a ring on a finger." In other cases, the Consorcio project was very complementary to the "interpersonal relations" training provided by a large World Bank project.[50]

- *The historical relationship between the health sector and the community.* In Carabayllo, CESIP would have had to work much longer and more intensively in this community to overcome the long-standing barriers of distrust. In contrast, there was a long history of cooperation between the Mothers' Clubs and the Health Center in Tarapoto, which helped make this one of the most successful experiences and facilitated the community women's inclusion in the multisectoral health committee.

- *The nature of the NGO's relationship with the community organizations and service providers.* In all of the Consorcio Mujer sites except Carabayllo, a long-standing relationship between the NGO, the women community leaders, and the health sector helped the NGO to play a catalytic role in setting terms and limits for the dialogue that were agreeable to all.

EPILOGUE AND FINAL REFLECTIONS

Consorcio Mujer did intensive work during 1999 to document the project's experiences, resulting in three publications.[51] These publications included an account of the experiences at each of the sites, as well as two training manuals—one each for providers and community health leaders on quality of care and users' rights.

While the NGOs and health centers involved in Consorcio Mujer all still exist, the consortium no longer officially exists. The organizations joined forces to design, raise funds for, and then implement the project. In the absence of a follow-up study, one can only hope that the people involved in these experiences—from each NGO, Health Center, and women's organization—took the lessons from experience and applied it to their continuing work. In one case, the advocacy component of the much more extensive Reprosalud project in Peru, is directed by one of the Consorcio NGOs—Movimiento Manuela Ramos. Reprosalud supports similar dialogue on quality of care between community women and health providers.

This study highlights the role of NGOs in effecting meaningful improvements in the quality of women's health care through facilitating community participation. Community oversight of quality of care in the provision of health services can be a delicate process; it is helpful to have an external entity managing it and monitoring the dynamics. The NGOs heard the views of both sides before bringing them together to engage in discussions and negotiation. Because users and providers speak different languages and operate from different places in the system, the NGOs played the role of mediator. The final Consorcio Mujer publication expresses concern about the sustainability of the dialogue process without this mediating influence. When aiming for systemic change, this points to the pitfalls of relying on NGOs, who mainly depend on short-term project funding to carry out their activities.

This study points to the effectiveness of Consorcio Mujer's strategy, which used a participatory process involving both users and providers to promote a system of health promotion based on citizenship and equality. An important element in the relative success of Consorcio Mujer's training strategy was that the participatory discussions and exercises led to the development of concrete proposals for improvements in service delivery and in actions to carry out the proposals. The combination of intensive interventions for attitude change, immediately followed by an opportunity to put these new principles into action, was a powerful change strategy.

LIST OF ORGANIZATIONS IN THE CONSORCIO MUJER PROJECT

LIMA

CESIP—Centro de Estudios Sociales y Publicaciones
    Lic. Silvia (Mina) Madalengoitia, Consorcio Mujer Project Director 1996–1999
    Ida Escudero—Coordinator of Project in Carabayllo

MOVIMIENTO MANUELA RAMOS
   Rocío Gutierrez, Coordinator of Project in San Juan de Miraflores
   Rosario Cardich, Consorcio Project Director from 1994–1996
   Fresia Carrasco, Representative to Technical Committee of Consorcio Mujer
CENTRO DE LA MUJER PERUANA FLORA TRISTÁN
   Ynga Villena, Coordinator of Project in San Juan de Lurigancho
   Ana Güezmes, Representative to Technical Committee of Consorcio Mujer

PIURA

CENTRO IDEAS
   Puente, Pilar (coordinator through 1997)
   Virginia Guero, Coordinator of Project in Salitral

CUSCO

AMAUTA—Centro de Estudios y Promoción de la Mujer
   Rosario Salazar, Project Coordinator

TARAPOTO

CEPCO—Centro de Estudios y Promoción Comunal del Oriente
   Maribel Becerril Ibérico, Project Coordinator.

NOTES

1. Most of the statistics in this section are cited to reflect the situation from 1995–2000, during and just after the implementation of the Consorcio Mujer project.

2. INEI, ENAHO 1995–1997 quoted in Ugarte and Monje 1999. "Lack of financial resources" could mean lack of funds to either pay the fees or travel costs.

3. United Nations 1995. "Core document forming part of the reports of states parties: Peru," submitted to the UN treaty bodies. HRI/CORE/1/Add.43/Rev1.

4. Ministerio de Salud and USAID 1997, 11. The rate has since fallen to 240, according to the Population Reference Bureau,, *Women of Our World*, 2002. There is much uncertainty about maternal mortality rates because of underreporting from rural areas. The WHO estimates for 2000 a rate of 410 for Peru, and gives 230 as the low end of the range of uncertainty; accessed on October 2005: http://www.who.int/reproductive-health/publications/maternal_mortality_2000/.

5. The "department" in Peru corresponds to the main regional subdivisions in government administration. The data in Figure 3.1 is drawn from Consorcio Mujer 1998.

6. Presidencia de la Republica, 1998, 18–19.

7. Alan Guttmacher Institute, 1994. Delicia Ferrando was the researcher for the Peru study. A more recent study of abortion in Peru by the same author is available: Ferrando, Delicia, *El Aborto Clandestino en el Perú*, Lima, Perú: Centro de la Mujer Peruana Flora Tristán and Pathfinder Internacional, 2002. The study of 2001 rates

estimates 352,000 abortions, an increase in the abortion rate per 100,000 live births from 43 to 54.

8. Data in Figure 3.2 is drawn from Consorcio Mujer 1998.

9. 1990–2000. It is now widely recognized within Peru that his government was authoritarian and corrupt, but in the mid-1990s, he enjoyed high favorability ratings for halting hyperinflation and defeating the Shining Path and MRTA terrorist organizations. He was driven out of office by election-rigging and corruption scandals in September 2000.

10. For more information on reform of the Peruvian health sector implemented under the Fujimori government, see Ugarte and Monje 1999. At the time of the author's visit to Peru in December 1998, the pilot phase of the health sector reform was in full swing in various departments, and coming soon in the others. The pilot efforts were mostly in health regions (which group together several departments) outside of Lima, and involved restructuring mid- and upper-level facilities into autonomous and mostly self-financed "networks and micro-networks." The author does not have updated (2005) information on this aspect of health sector reform.

11. Unfortunately, the bibliography of the Consorcio Mujer publications does not include most of these studies, which were evaluation reports. The author was familiar with the studies during the 1990s, because discussion of their findings was part of the process of negotiating the grant to Consorcio Mujer to conduct a quality of care evaluation. One is cited in Consorcio Mujer 1998: MINSA, HAMA, OPS 1993. "Evaluación de las Condiciones de Eficiencia de los Servicios y Programas Materno Infantiles y Transmisibles."

12. See Center for Reproductive Rights and CLADEM 1998 for a study of human rights abuses in the health system in the mid-1990s.

13. This emphasis was driven by the almost exclusive use of couple years of protection (CYPs) as the outcome indicator for USAID's family planning programs in the late 1980s and early 1990s. Long-acting methods give multiple years of protection, making the "cost per CYP" much lower than for provision of oral contraceptives or condoms, for example. In visits to Peru in 1992 and 1993, the author met with representatives of Pathfinder International and USAID. At that time, Pathfinder's program concentrated almost solely on IUD provision.

14. He dissolved the Congress, and then called a constitutional assembly controlled by those loyal to his party.

15. The Basic Health and Nutrition Project funded by the World Bank conducted community-based needs assessments, for which they contracted feminist NGOs. Project 2000, funded by USAID with Pathfinder International, aimed to raise the quality of care and user satisfaction in many services where it intervened. Most notably, Reprosalud, a USAID-funded $19 million project was awarded in 1994 to one of the largest feminist NGOs in Peru—Movimiento Manuela Ramos—to implement on a massive scale in low-income provinces a model community participation program in reproductive health and credit programs for women.

16. See Chapter 2 for a fuller discussion of how the Peruvian NGO networks met this challenge.

17. Many health workers were "contracted" as opposed to civil service ("de planta") employees, and were hired with specific productivity goals. If these were not met, they could be fired, or transferred to an undesirable location.

18. The Consorcio Mujer members involved in this project included Movimiento Manuela Ramos, Centro de la Mujer Peruana Flora Tristán, and Centro de Estudios Sociales y Publicaciones (CESIP) in Lima; Centro de Estudios y Promoción de la Mujer Amauta in the Andean highlands; Centro IDEAS in the rural coast zone; and Centro de Estudios y Promoción Comunal del Oriente in the Amazon region. The Ford Foundation supported the project in two grants: the first of $100,000 and the second of $182,000, with a third grant in 1999 to produce the final publications. The Consorcio was formed in order to carry out this project, and was dissolved after the production of the publications in 2000.

19. The exception was CESIP's project in Carabayllo, a municipality in Lima. The outcomes reflected this difference, with less success in the dialogue between the community and the health providers.

20. Rosario Cardich of Movimiento Manuela Ramos directed Phase One of the project, and Silvia Madalengoitia of CESIP directed Phase Two.

21. From Consorcio Mujer's educational brochure for women leaders.

22. Hola and Portugal, 1997.

23. Except when indicated otherwise, the quotes in this study are from abridged transcripts of taped interviews during the author's 1998 visit to the six project sites.

24. Judith Bruce, "Fundamental elements of the quality of care: A simple framework," *Studies in Family* Planning 21, No. 2 (1990).

25. Drawn from Consorcio Mujer's educational leaflet for women leaders: "Let's Be Citizens, not Patients."

26. Such questions proved much more productive than asking a general question about a client's level of satisfaction, the answers to which tended to indicate falsely high levels of satisfaction.

27. All of these findings are summarized from Consorcio Mujer 1998.

28. Ibid., 42.

29. The committees, organized in the mid-1990s with the encouragement of the Ministry of Health, included representatives from the health sector, other ministries, municipal officials, NGOs, and, occasionally, community organizations. The ministry hoped that by institutionalizing such communication, the resources of all institutions active in health promotion in one geographic area could be directed toward common goals and strategies.

30. The author attended this meeting.

31. The Rural Women's Network was an organization of peasant women in the Piura area with district level subnetworks of more than 1,000 women.

32. In the decentralization scheme, each network might include the maternity hospitals, health centers, and health posts in a health region. The institution designated as the coordinator of the network was in a key position to implement new programs and guidelines.

33. Consorcio Mujer 1998.

34. The levels of intimidation of users differed among the six project sites, depending on provincial fertility rates and on the willingness of regional, subregional, and health center directors to resist pressures from higher-ups. When a midwife was under intense pressure to meet her monthly quota of sterilizations, she

in turn would exert substantial pressure on women. One United Nations professional described how in one village she visited, Quechua women fled into the hills whenever the public health midwife came to their village, because her pressures made them afraid of being coerced into being sterilized.

35. The sterilization campaigns ended abruptly in January 1998 when Giulia Tamayo of CLADEM Peru, a women's rights network, exposed related human rights abuses in the media; see CLADEM 1999.

36. There was widespread migration to Lima and other cities from the Quechua-speaking highlands in the 1990s; some were refugees from armed conflicts between terrorists and government troops. Others migrated for economic reasons.

37. Some health officials interviewed would not admit that fees are used to supplement salaries, while others confirmed that doing so is a widespread, but unofficial, practice. Health professionals interviewed in this study also pointed out that user fees are an incentive to improve quality, since attracting more users brings more income to the health service.

38. According to many informants in the Consorcio Mujer program, and in the Reprosalud project in the Andean highlands—from the author's interviews with staff and women leaders involved during the mid-term evaluation in 2002.

39. Quotes are from Consorcio Mujer 1998.

40. The health system in Peru, in concert with many international NGOs, has long trained community health promoters to carry out specific health promotion tasks in the community. These promoters are usually not paid for their time, or reimbursed for expenses.

41. The new General Health Law was passed in July 1997. Consorcio Mujer trainers gave participants in both workshop groups a poster with a list of users' rights as established by the law.

42. The training manuals were published in limited quantities. The participating NGOs and the author have copies.

43. Consorcio Mujer, 1998. This is an interchange documented during the 1994 evaluation.

44. The content of the following section is taken solely from the author's interviews in the six sites.

45. From interview with Centro Ideas staff in 1998.

46. From interview with Silvia Madalengoitia in 1998.

47. The one exception was an implementation failure. In San Juan de Lurigancho, the training by Centro Flora Tristán took place before the Consorcio had completed the modules, and the process was not the same as in the other sites.

48. This exception was Tarapoto, and may be due to methodology failure; it was the only site where the interview with the users' group was in a multisectoral committee meeting with health providers present.

49. Unfortunately, since Consorcio Mujer was a project that ended in 1999, carrying out a follow-up study would be difficult.

50. The Basic Health and Nutrition Project (*Proyecto de Salud y Nutrición Básica*).

51. See three Consorcio Mujer publications from the year 2000 in the bibliography.

4

CONVERSATIONS AND CONTROVERSIES: A SEXUALITY EDUCATION PROGRAM IN CHILE

The confidence placed in me is a thousand times more valuable than what I contributed. I have grown, and I have changed. . . . I loved it that you all believed in us and gave us responsibility. (Student facilitator in Chilean sex education program—JOCAS)

INTRODUCTION

Although there has long been worldwide support and united political will to protect the health of infants and small children, this strong consensus erodes as children grow up. The seemingly universal adult instinct to protect "innocent" infants and young children falters in adolescence[1] when the major health threats stem from unprotected sexual activity inside and outside of marriage, early childbearing, depression, physical and sexual violence, unsafe abortion, substance abuse, and risk-taking behavior leading to accidents.[2]

All over the world, sexually active young people are denied their rights to the education and services they need to protect their health because of controversies occurring at all levels, from the United Nations summits to individual families. Issues of adolescent sexual and reproductive health stirred fierce polemics at the 1999 and 2004 United Nations post-ICPD meetings[3] and the United Nations General Assembly Special Session on the Child in May 2002.[4] As with the abortion issue, this "hot-button" topic threatened to derail efforts to reach a consensus before the final documents were signed.

These controversies focus on young people's right to the means to prevent pregnancy and infection if they are sexually active. One side argues that providing education and services implicitly condones youths' sexual activity and undermines parental authority.[5] The other side argues that states have the obligation to provide adolescents with information and services on reproduction and sexuality to protect their health, no matter whether their parents approve. In myriad local, national, and global debates, decision-makers cannot agree on giving the health needs and rights of young people higher priority than the opinions of parents or socially conservative pressure groups.

Most young people are politically disenfranchised; in most countries, those under 18 cannot vote and have no official means of political participation to defend their interests. As a result, young people have great difficulty gaining access to the resources they need —for health, education and employment— without adult support. For this reason, the literature in the adolescent sexual and reproductive health (ASRH) field speaks of adults as "gatekeepers." A human rights framework, however, refers to adults in local and national governments—in the policy environment of the young—as "duty-bearers," that is those with the *obligation* to protect and promote the health and development of young people. These adults do not just keep the gate; they are obliged to open it when young people's lives and well-being are at stake.

Adults with responsibilities for young people either at the family or policy level often are ambivalent about sexual and reproductive health programs. As a result, they fail to fulfill their obligations to the young, and programs and policies may become mired in controversy and bureaucratic infighting. Because many necessary and excellent programs never see the light of day or die a slow death after a brief success, the worldwide supply of reproductive and sexual health education and services for youth is woefully insufficient.

Box 4.1
Adolescents' Right to Sexual and Reproductive Health Education and Services

States should provide adolescents with safe and supportive environments where they can participate in decisions that affect their health, build life skills, acquire appropriate information, receive counselling and be able to negotiate the health behavior choices they make. The realization of the right to health of adolescents is dependent on the development of youth-sensitive health care, which respects confidentiality and privacy and includes appropriate sexual and reproductive health services. (Committee on Economic Social and Cultural Rights, General Comment #14 on the right to the highest attainable standard of health)[6]

This failure to protect the health of the young is widespread in the predominantly Catholic countries of Latin America.

This study analyzes one of these brief successes: a nationwide sexuality education program in Chile. From 1996 through 2000 the Chilean government promoted the "Conversation Workshops on Relationships and Sexuality," best known in Chile by their acronym in Spanish: *JOCAS.*[7] (A slightly different version of the same methodology based in communities, rather than schools, and called *JOCCAS,* was also part of the initiative.) Despite a sharply polarized sociocultural environment on issues of sexuality and reproduction, the program's innovative design enabled it to sidestep the initial controversy and be implemented massively.

Initially developed for use within the schools, the JOCAS are a three-part series of highly participatory workshops involving the whole school community: students, teachers, administrators, and parents. As a participatory, decentralized program without a standardized curriculum, the JOCAS model was politically feasible for a socially conservative environment. It had powerful effects in breaking down taboos against conversations on sensitive subjects and was remarkable for its emphasis on the autonomous learning and empowerment of adolescents, as well as its relative simplicity and low cost of implementation. The main disadvantage of the model is that its design does not guarantee young participants access to complete and comprehensive information on sexuality and reproductive health. Furthermore, as will be seen, the program's initial success in side-stepping controversy did not continue. Eventually, sexuality education requires a commitment to diversity of opinion and the defense of young people's well-being that is likely to entail considerable political costs for its proponents.

Just as the Consorcio Mujer program in Peru promoted women's participation in health sector services, the JOCAS promoted greater student participation in at least one aspect of their schooling. The JOCAS were part of a broader democratization effort in Chilean society and in the schools. This movement promoted participatory teaching methods to encourage less authoritarian dynamics in the relationship between teachers and students and to increase student achievement. Participatory mechanisms such as student and parent councils were also encouraged.

The study analyzes how the political, cultural, and multisectoral dynamics surrounding sexuality education affected the program and led to compromises that not only denied young people their right to free expression but also eventually debilitated the popular program by saddling it with the stigma of polemic and undermining political support for its continuance. The JOCAS experience also reveals how seemingly trivial changes in program design can empower or disempower the young participants. The lessons from this experience are particularly relevant today as sexuality education programs for young people are under attack in many countries.

SEXUALITY EDUCATION IN CHILE

In Chile, much of the concern over adolescent pregnancy stems from the growing numbers of unmarried adolescents having children. At the time the JOCAS program was developed in 1995, an often-quoted figure from the 1992 Chilean census[8] was that 40,000 babies were born to adolescent mothers per year, 85.7 percent of them single. Although the fertility rate among fifteen- to nineteen-year-olds is midrange by Latin American standards[9] and has remained stable during the 1980s and 1990s, the rates for those aged fifteen to seventeen increased dramatically in the same period while the rates for those aged eighteen and nineteen fell. The percentage of these births corresponding to single women rose from 40 percent in 1980 to 77 percent in 1998.

While demographic data graphically illustrate the problem, the political and social climate is not conducive to addressing it. Chile is known for being a socially conservative country. Until 2004, Chile was one of two countries in the world where divorce was still illegal.[10] Abortion is not legal even to save the mother's life.

During the seventeen years of the military dictatorship from 1973 to 1990, the social conservatism of the country's military rulers—with roots in the premodern oligarchy—transformed Chile from one of the most liberal Latin American countries to one of the most socially conservative.[11] Although the advent of democracy in 1990 relaxed some aspects of official policy, most sexual and reproductive health policies remain relatively restrictive. The Catholic Church wields a great deal of political influence in Chile, more so than in any other Latin American country, in part due to its progressive role during the dictatorship in defending human rights and social justice.[12] Therefore, it was hardly surprising that in the first year of the *Concertación* government in 1990, initiatives to address unwanted adolescent pregnancies ran into political obstacles.

However, there were some important advances. First, the incoming government established the National Commission on AIDS (CONASIDA),

Table 4.1
Changes in Adolescent Fertility in Chile 1980–1998

Year	Mother's Age and Adolescent Fertility Rate (AFR)		
	15 years	16 years	17 years
1980	13	33	59
1998	23	50	71

Source: Instituto Nacional de Estatísticas, Estadísticas Vitales.
Note: AFR is number of live births for each 1,000 women in the age group.

and growing consciousness of the emerging epidemic added some impetus to initiatives to provide sexuality education to young people in Chile. Second, Chile signed the Convention on the Rights of the Child, and Congress ratified it in September 1990.[13] States that sign the Convention must bring their policies and programs into line with its terms, including protection for adolescents' health through family planning services.[14] Third, the government revoked a policy barring pregnant young women and young mothers from the daytime public school program.[15]

This last decree stirred the Ministry of Education to address the issue of unwanted adolescent pregnancies among schoolgirls. In 1991 the Ministry of Education (MINEDUC), under the leadership of Education Minister Ricardo Lagos and María de la Luz Silva, director of MINEDUC's Women's Program, convened a "consultative committee" to formulate a national policy on sex education.[16] The committee included representatives from the Ministry of Health, CONASIDA, the National Women's Service (SERNAM), prominent NGOs, academics, human rights groups, Catholic and Masonic groups, UNFPA, and a progressive Catholic theologian. The committee represented very diverse viewpoints but agreed on a common agenda of values: respect for human rights and dignity; responsibility toward others; self-esteem and self-respect; and promotion of attitudes of solidarity, acceptance, and love for others. The committee also recognized the sharp cultural and political divisions in Chilean society on promotion of young people's sexual and reproductive health and agreed to devise a policy that would respect this diversity of opinion. "They [the Committee] realized that it would not be possible to implement a centralized sex education program."[17] It reached a consensus that sex education programs would be completely decentralized and that each establishment would develop its own institutional program involving administrators, teachers, students and parents. "Considering that . . . it is impossible to incorporate a common discourse into the school curriculum, a mechanism is required that decentralizes all decisions regarding issues in which diverse norms, values and beliefs exist."[18]

Not everyone agreed with the decision to decentralize.[19] While decentralization was useful politically in that it enabled a sexuality education program to go forward, the decision to leave decisions on content to each individual school did not universally guarantee young people access to all the relevant information. However, the committee's recommendation of decentralized, participatory approaches is consistent with a trend in modern democracies. In addition, since Chilean law provides schools with considerable autonomy, reinforced by the military dictatorship in the last year of its rule,[20] a more centralized approach would have been difficult to enforce. The central political tension between a decentralized, participatory, school-by-school approach and a human rights framework with universal guarantees of children's rights was resolved in favor of the former. One result was that no specific content could be mandated by government authorities.

Two years later in 1993, after receiving feedback from schools and a variety of stakeholders around the country, the Ministry of Education released its official Sexuality Education Policy. In early 1994, soon after the election of President Eduardo Frei and the assumption of a new cabinet, the "Multisectoral Committee on Sex Education and Prevention of Adolescent Pregnancy"[21] was convened, comprised of representatives from the Education, Health and Women's ministries, and the National AIDS Commission, along with UNFPA and the National Youth Institute (INJ). The Ministry of Education in 1995 contracted EDUK, a Chilean educational NGO, to run five pilot projects using the JOCAS methodology[22] within the framework of its new policy. Participation by the schools was voluntary, and MINEDUC offered training and technical assistance.

The implementation went very well and excited enthusiasm among the participants as well as education ministry officials and staff.[23] In the school-based version, the JOCAS are comprised of a series of three workshops, known as "moments," involving the entire school community in conversations—students, administrators, teachers, and parents. These three workshops completely interrupt the school's routine for two hours. (See the following section for a full description.) The JOCAS were designed to fit in with the school reform program known as "MECE Media," which proposed to "transform the high-school into a space that interprets students' preferences and interests," to foster "greater ongoing student participation...in project design, execution, and evaluation," and to "open up the school to the community."[24]

In 1996 the Ministry of Education trained its regional staff to assume responsibility for forty more JOCAS in three provinces and sponsored two evaluations of these experiences.[25] Despite the fierce controversies that arose, JOCAS were scaled up significantly in 1997 and were held in more than 200 schools. In 1998 and 1999 the demand for JOCAS from the schools was so great that MINEDUC's budget could not cover all the requests.[26] By early 2000, the ministry had implemented JOCAS in roughly 600 schools nationwide, more than half of the high schools in the country.

It is a testament to the ability of this model to operate in socially polarized environments that the JOCAS were the second most popular initiative of the Chilean government during these four years.[27] They received the official approval of the Chilean Catholic bishops' conference in 1998. The level and speed with which MINEDUC scaled up the program was impressive. The government's ability to do so probably stemmed from several factors: the program's high-level ministerial and multisectoral support; the decentralized principle of local control mandated by the 1993 guidelines; favorable findings from the initial evaluations; the inclusion of parents and community services in the program; a simple yet well-designed training manual and training program; and the voluntary and participatory nature of the

JOCAS model. According to most informants, the program enjoyed a remarkably high level of acceptance and popularity.

Nonetheless, the government eventually discontinued the program. When a new administration took office in 2000, support for JOCAS was reduced to the presence of a manual on the MINEDUC web site, even though the new president was none other than Ricardo Lagos, the former education minister who had initiated the entire process.[28] The gradual undermining of the JOCAS shows how traditional cultural and political elites were able to counter the overwhelming popular enthusiasm for sexuality education for young people. The widespread acceptance of an educational strategy that avoided monolithic moral or ethical positions on sexuality was not sufficient to counteract the pressures from the Catholic Church hierarchy and the conservative media.

THE JOCAS PROGRAM MODEL

Description of the Goals and Methodology

The JOCAS [29] are a decentralized and participatory educational program with three main aims:

- to break the taboo on talking about sex and sexual relationships, initiating conversations on these topics;
- to put the school community in touch with services and professionals in the surrounding community who can respond to the needs of youth in these areas; and
- to empower participants—especially adolescents—to use these conversations to gather information, analyze common problems and identify the best courses of action.

During the preparatory phase an organizing committee of administrators, teachers, students, and parents is trained to run the JOCAS' three- to two-hour sessions, which take place on separate days.

First workshop: talking it over and generating questions. Led by a trained peer facilitator, small groups of no more than twenty students meet for one to two hours and talk in an unstructured way about relationships and sexuality. In a large school, this workshop can involve as many as thirty groups of students meeting simultaneously. The teachers and parents meet separately for their own conversations while community resource people unobtrusively observe the small groups. Speaking from their experiences, participants raise their doubts and concerns and share knowledge. At the end of the exercise, each group summarizes its concerns in the form of questions. After the first workshop, the resource people and the school's organizing committee review the questions and discuss possible responses. This initial experience is designed to engage both the emotional and rational sides of the participants and to awaken their interest in learning more.

Second workshop: gaining knowledge and insight. In the second workshop, the resource people meet with groups of students of the same age to answer the questions raised in the first workshop. There is also time for dialogue. These adults represent three areas of expertise: health professionals, psychologists or social workers, and religious leaders or other respected figures who can address "values." The goal is for participants to incorporate new knowledge and perspectives, to enrich their reflections on relationships and sexuality, and to put the students directly in touch with people in their community who can provide further services.

Third workshop: discerning options. The final workshop has two stages. In the first, participants return to their first discussion groups, which then choose a previously discussed problematic situation and imagine themselves in the role of its different protagonists (parents, boyfriend, girlfriend). They then discuss at least three different ways to resolve the problem. The aim is not to arrive at a consensus but to help members reflect on their options. Once this discussion is finished, the students from each age group meet with the participating parents from each grade to share the outcome of their discussions. In the original model, the dialogue with parents did not take place.

Celebrating the experience. In the original model the student, parent, and teacher groups created murals and skits, followed by a celebration of the experience. However, the young people's artistic expressions on sexual topics proved too controversial, and murals were eliminated. In the current model, the mixed parent/student groups and the teacher/administrator groups prepare skits, songs, and poems for the celebration.

The Theory of Learning and Discernment

The JOCAS are based on ideas about health education in which the learner acquires the motivation to learn and the skills to make informed, autonomous decisions. As one of the main JOCAS designers said: "People not only have the right to information; they have the right to learn, which is quite different." [30]

A key objective of the JOCAS[31] is that young people learn new information and life skills. The model recognizes the informal origins of most learning about relationships and sexuality, and it activates informal conversations and information-seeking as the most effective mode of learning. With regard to learning life skills, the theory of pedagogy and social change underlying the JOCAS is that mutually respectful and uncensored conversations among peers—in which questions and problems are aired and different options for action are analyzed—will strengthen the ability of each participant to "*discern*" or identify the behavior and actions that best fit his or her values and goals.

Operating in the highly complex realm of sexuality and relationships where strong feelings and sensations often overpower judgment, the model gives central importance to *discernment*—defined as the thought process underlying sound decision-making—as a key life skill for young people, along with communication and negotiation. Breaking the taboo on conversation helps participants put emotions and sensations into words, thus enabling them to negotiate needs and desires with others openly.

Given the emphasis on discernment and decision-making, the JOCAS explicitly adopt a conception of morality that gives highest priority to individual autonomy and the person's conscience, as opposed to the traditional morality of sacred, fixed norms.[32] This clash in philosophies was at the root of much of the conservative opposition to the JOCAS. The president of the education section of the Chilean Bishopric (*Episcopado*), Francisco Javier Cox, expressed the opponents' point of view:[33]

If you have a 16-year-old listen to people who tell him different things, he becomes completely disoriented. Where is the truth that he seeks? If he receives a kaleidoscope of opinions, he says to himself, "Well, if it's all the same, I'll do what seems best to me." This is just throwing information at him, not educating him. The JOCAS can cause distortions without a framework of values. Maybe later the boy will choose another path, but when he is still developing one cannot put a lot of options in front of him and just let him decide.[34]

Finally, the JOCAS are designed to have a ripple effect, referred to as *resonance* by the program's designers. In the theory underlying the JOCAS, increasing young people's ability to converse on these topics is a key outcome of the model and has multiple effects. The workshops are designed to inspire more and better conversations among peers, within the school community, and in families long after the JOCAS take place.

The JOCAS' Democratizing Influence

Many participants remarked on the intense, emotional effect of the experience within each school and on many of the participants.[35] The widespread enthusiasm for this program among school communities, municipalities, NGOs, and ministry officials speaks to the power of involving every sector of the school or community in horizontal conversations on matters that deeply affect the lives of all human beings.

Several observers mentioned that the period of dictatorship affected all social institutions and stifled participation. In a country in transition from a seventeen-year dictatorship, grassroots models like the JOCAS unleash much pent-up energy and democratizing impulses, both within schools and in communities. Within the relatively top-down didactic culture of traditional schools, the JOCAS were a breath of fresh air. One student's testimony is typical: "The confidence placed in me is a thousand times more valuable than what I contributed. I have grown and I have changed. . . . I loved it that you all believed in us and gave us responsibility."[36]

Dr. Raquel Child, director of the Chilean government's National AIDS Commission (CONASIDA) during the period of the JOCAS, described their democratizing influence:

This model does not involve an official governmental discourse . . . but rather people's own words, meanings, emotions, difficulties and problems. The lack of an official discourse or agenda . . . is an important advance from the perspective of democracy and capacity building. One of the strengths of the JOCAS design is that they rely on local implementation teams so that the model devolves technical skills and responsibility to the community. . . . This methodology is applicable to any topic.[37]

Part of the democratizing influence of the JOCAS was their enhancement of free expression. The taboo on speaking about sexuality was broken simultaneously for adults and students alike, and the conversations often felt revolutionary to the participants. Although official evaluations did not set out to measure this enhancement of free expression and horizontal interactions, numerous testimonials bear witness to the catalytic power of the program.

I think the JOCAS can be a true turning point in the life of a school, that there are ripple effects for other issues, and that the experience can even change the way the school is governed. . . . Because this affects us all, [talking about] the issue changes [each individual] as well. . . . This is why the model is so powerful. No one leaves a JOCAS unchanged.[38]

EVALUATION OF THE JOCAS: EXPECTATIONS AND RESULTS

The JOCAS were intended to have the following measurable results:

- increase young people's access to correct information to protect their health;
- increase their access to services;
- improve their communications, negotiations and decision-making skills; and
- improve and increase young people's connections with adults.

While all these goals were important, most evaluations of the model focused on increases in the number of conversations and improvement in their quality as perceived by all the actors involved. For the most part, they did not measure increases in knowledge or in service use. However, as part of the inquiry about conversations, most measured information-seeking behavior by students and evaluated the connections with parents and teachers.

Using the frameworks for adolescent health promotion developed by WHO, UNFPA, and UNICEF,[39] the following table (Table 4.2) illustrates how the JOCAS were designed to meet the requirements for successful adolescent health programs. The second column notes the successes and failures identified in this study and in the evaluations carried out by SERNAM and the Ministry of Education.[40]

The evaluations of the 1996 and 1997 JOCAS[41] show both high levels of satisfaction among the participants and effectiveness in impact on the quantity and quality of conversations following the JOCAS among the youth, as well as between youth and the adults in their lives. EDUK conducted a follow-up survey of thirty-six schools involved in the 1996 JOCAS twelve to eighteen months after the event;[42] another study contracted by the Ministry of Education used a sample of 117 schools in the 1997 JOCAS.[43]

EDUK evaluated the JOCAS for impact in three areas: increase in the quantity and quality of conversations on relationship and sexuality topics among students, teachers, and parents (the main expected result); the institutionalization of school-based curriculum or activities related to these topics; and increased institutional networks in the surrounding communities to increase availability of information, counseling, and health services for students.

The MINEDUC study evaluated the JOCAS for later effects in five areas: quantity of conversations, quality of conversations, available information, impact on STIs, and impact on adolescent pregnancy.[44]

Although not explicitly studied as an indicator in the surveys, one of the most important results of the JOCAS mentioned by all informants was that the participating adults "had their blindfolds removed" with regard to the level of the students' sexual activity. These new realizations of the students' needs for information, counseling and services were expected to create emotional momentum among the adults in the school community—school administrators, teachers, and parents—to implement continuing sexuality education programs.

The clearest and most favorable results of the JOCAS are in the area of more and better conversations on sexuality. In the EDUK evaluation, all categories of respondents reported that students asked more questions and sought more information. Seventy-nine percent of teachers and students reported an increase in conversations on relationships and sexuality. In both evaluations, slightly more than half the students said that they perceived a more positive emotional climate surrounding these issues in conversations with teachers. The student focus groups clarified the nature of this change: previous references to sexuality tended to be either "pornographic" or in the form of jokes; the subject could not be discussed respectfully and seriously.

"The JOCAS triggered an environment in which [resource people and teachers] were seeking training and asking questions. Thousands of people ask questions during the JOCAS."[45] The program theory posits that this experience is catalytic, leading to increased motivation to keep asking

Table 4.2
Analysis of the Results of the JOCAS

Requirements for Successful Adolescent Health Promotion	Successes and Failures in the Expected Outcomes in Practice (Expected Outcomes in Italics, Comments on the Experience in Normal Font)
1. Youth acquire accurate information.	*The second workshop in which community resource people respond to the questions of the students is the first opportunity to acquire information.* In general, the JOCAS fulfilled this expectation, and most evaluations show a high appreciation for this workshop. However, there were few mechanisms for quality control of the information provided by the local resource people, and some schools censored certain topics.
	Ministry of Education officials noted that many schools established ongoing sexuality education programs after the JOCAS but had no systematic data on this question.
	One expected outcome is that youth seek additional information after the JOCAS. The evaluation showed this outcome to be the most notable success, with students reporting more information-seeking post-JOCAS, approaching both teachers and other sources with their questions.
	Young people's access to additional information is higher in the JOCCAS[a] through the community resource fair run by health institutions, other government agencies and local NGOs.
2. Youth acquire life skills (negotiation, conflict resolution, critical thinking, decision-making, and communication).[b]	*The discernment exercise in the third workshop and conversations about issues should lead to improved ability to communicate on these topics and to weigh different options, which in turn should lead to decision-making that promotes health.*
	Fully 85 percent of evaluation respondents reported an improved ability to discuss these topics. There is no evidence about other behavioral changes because of the JOCAS.
	Content analysis of some of the conversations in the JOCAS showed many thoughtful and rich discussions of the different options for action in a problematic situation. However, evaluators also noted a problem with the quality of some conversations when the student facilitator who led the group imposed a judgmental and morally rigid social norm, thus closing off discussion.[c]
3. Youth obtain counseling (especially	*Breaking the silence on these topics with parents and teachers should make these adults more accessible for counseling. New connections with community resource people might provide new counselors.*

144

during crises) and have a connection with at least one supportive adult.	In the 1996 and 1997 JOCAS evaluations, 50 percent of students reported a positive effect on conversations with teachers, while even more noted a positive effect on conversations among peers. While parental participation was very low, in the small sub-sample whose parents (mainly mothers) attended, students noted positive effects on their conversations. The evaluation showed no increased connections with the community resource people after the JOCAS.
4. Youth have access to health services, including those for reproductive health.	*The health provider who participates in the JOCAS (usually a midwife) should establish herself in the young people's minds as a sympathetic adult and a resource, thus encouraging them to come for services if they need them. An expected benefit was that the students would seek out the social workers or the midwife who attended the JOCAS later if they had additional needs for information or services.* Because of political controversies regarding adolescents' access to contraceptives without parental consent, increase in young people's usage of confidential reproductive health services was never an explicit, public goal of the JOCAS. In addition, increased usage was never included in the evaluations due to turf divisions: MINEDUC would not set a goal for and evaluate health services that do not fall under its jurisdiction.
5. Youth live in a safe, supportive environment.	*The JOCAS dialogues between teachers and students, and those between parents and students, were designed to create more supportive inter-generational dialogue and more support for sexuality education.* Fifty-two percent of participants noted a positive change in the emotional climate surrounding the issues. See other comments in #3 on increased adult-young person communications. Finally, teachers and administrators reported that the JOCAS were a stimulus to learning more about participatory pedagogical methods, a favorable byproduct in the hierarchical culture of the traditional public school.
6. Youth have opportunities for participating meaningfully in their communities and in programs and policies to promote their health.	*Student leaders participate fully in the planning of the JOCAS and are trained to lead small-group discussions in the first and third workshops. Many informants found this aspect of the JOCAS very important. Having students be entirely in charge of running the first and third workshops without adult supervision was entirely unprecedented in most schools. The orderly fashion in which the students led and organized these workshops was astonishing to many of the teachers and administrators.* Some interviewees asserted that students' protagonism in the school-based JOCAS was reduced after public controversies arose in 1996.

---

[a]JOCCAS are the community-based version of the school-based JOCAS. Previous drafts of this chapter discussed the differences between JOCAS and JOCCAS in some depth, and are available from the author.

[b]The enumeration of the "life skills" identified as protective factors for adolescent health comes from UNICEF, UNAIDS, WHO, 2002, 29.

[c]Notes from conversation with Irma Palma and Paula Arriagada, September 2002.

questions and keep learning. However, only 35 to 45 percent of adult respondents reported an improved climate in conversations among adults.

In some cases JOCAS may have contributed toward a more democratic and horizontal relationship between teachers and students. Several other informants testified to the adults' surprise at how maturely the students behaved and conversed on these subjects.

One of the main strengths of the methodology is that it gives the young people a space that they use freely and positively, which produces a great impact in adults' perception of the students' behavior.[46]

I am impressed by the good conduct of my fellow students. They behaved better than they do in classes. Even the worst troublemakers were calm. . . . For me, it was an extremely important experience because for the first time I had the opportunity to find out that I like being a leader. *Student coordinator*[47]

I discovered that I am no longer so ashamed to talk in public; I even like it. I believe I have more self-confidence now. I brought out into the open the personality that I had hidden away. *Student facilitator*

The MINEDUC evaluation found the organizational benefits to be mainly "integration within the school," that is, improved relations between teachers and students or new opportunities for democratic participation in the schools (51 percent). The evaluation likewise noted the JOCAS' "stimulus to the school community in other areas" (57 percent) and an incentive for teachers to learn new pedagogical methods. The EDUK evaluation found that 41 percent of the schools had adapted the JOCAS methodology to other topics, often substance abuse prevention programs.

Both evaluations indicate that there was only a slight increase in integration of sexuality education into the curriculum. In the MINEDUC evaluation, 85 percent of schools already had "some activity related to relationships and sexuality"[48]—mostly basic reproduction information in biology class—but the teachers highlighted the participatory methodology as a highly valued innovation.

Fathers, mothers, students, and teachers in the focus groups perceived the positive effects fade without sustained follow-up interventions. Repeatedly, focus group participants wondered about the continuity of JOCAS and proposed to include younger students in them.[49] Figure 4.1 from the MINEDUC evaluation[50] showed the significantly different needs of each sector. Sixty-two percent of students stated that their main need was information while only 25 to 29 percent of the adults concurred. Parents and students gave similar priority to human relations (44 percent and 52 percent), while the majority of teachers were eager to be better trained in the new participatory methodologies. It is ironic, given the Catholic Church's insistence on involvement of parents to ensure attention to values, that few of the parents surveyed wanted or expected the school to impart values in sexuality education.

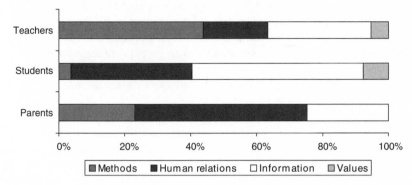

Figure 4.1
Needs Assessment: Opinions of Parents, Teachers, and Students

Many expected the experience of the JOCAS to stimulate the school to hold similar exercises every year. Although there is no concrete data on repeat JOCAS in succeeding years, some evidence exists that autonomous replications were still widespread in 2003, four years after the ministry stopped promoting the program.[51]

Since the existing evaluations were all based on retrospective data collection on perceptions of impact, no clear association can be drawn between the JOCAS and decreases in levels of unwanted pregnancies or STIs or increases in the adolescents' use of health services. However, the JOCAS program coincided with the establishment of adolescent health services by MENSAL, and these services were introduced to the JOCAS participants.

Obstacles to Parental Involvement

The JOCAS rarely met the goal of improving communications between parents and children even though everyone insisted that this was a goal of the exercise. A number of factors led to this failure to achieve parental involvement precisely at the time when the issue of parental authority became a lightning rod in the political controversy surrounding the JOCAS.

While there were many points of contention in the multisectoral commission that set the guidelines for sexuality education in Chile in the early 1990s, all agreed that parental participation was essential. The designers and supporters of the original model of the JOCAS—most of whom fall into the "liberal" or "secular" end of the spectrum—were in full agreement and built parental involvement into the program. For this reason, the organizing committee is comprised of the entire "school community," which explicitly includes parents. They are also invited to participate in the JOCAS by holding group discussions among themselves in the first workshop and participating in the third and final workshop with students.

Those in charge of the JOCAS within the Ministry of Education wrestled with the challenge of securing parental involvement and acknowledged this aspect as a shortcoming of the program: "The process of involving parents has been extremely slow. Less than a third of parents come; generally, it is a small group of mothers. In fact, it is mainly the young people who hold conversations."[52] Most informants and all evaluations agreed that fathers rarely attended the JOCAS.

Not surprisingly, the effects on family life were limited to those few parents who attended, and young people expressed sharp dissatisfaction with their absence in the evaluations.[53] For those parents who did attend, the benefits in communication were confirmed by the students and parents interviewed. The JOCAS vividly demonstrated to the adults the communications gap between parents and children and the high cost of not having conversations about sexuality.[54]

Since parental involvement was such a high priority for all involved—conservatives and liberals, ministry officials and students—why was participation so low? Several answers emerge from the evaluations.

One commonly cited obstacle to parental involvement was logistical: parents who work full-time could not attend during the school day. The 1995 pilots experimented with several strategies, including holding a "sharing" meeting on a Saturday after the JOCAS were over. However, none of their strategies worked, suggesting that other factors besides employment limited parental participation. In desperation, one school held a JOCAS just for parents at the compulsory annual meeting when grades are given out.[55]

Another reason cited for low parental participation was the active opposition of some fathers who tried to prevent the mothers from attending.[56] Some said that their wives already knew the information, while others were afraid that their wives would be asked to share information about their sexual life.[57]

EDUK also identified traditional gender roles that assign the woman sole responsibility for the education of children as an underlying factor in paternal resistance or indifference. Mothers generally represent the family at most parent meetings in the schools on any topic. According to a father in one focus group, "Very few of us fathers dare to show up at the school to see what is going on with our children."[58]

Yet there are deeper, more systemic answers to this question of why this key component of the program did not work as expected, having to do with the school system itself. Worldwide, secondary schools have had great difficulty in involving parents meaningfully in important events and decisions in the life of the school,[59] and the Chilean school system is no exception. Parents and guardians distance themselves from the schools as their children grow older, due to the greater autonomy of adolescents and the complex organization of most secondary schools. Another barrier is geographic. Secondary schools tend to draw students from a larger area than primary schools, and as a result, many families live a considerable distance away.

In addition, specific historical factors related to the organizational culture of Chilean schools may help explain parents' relative exclusion from secondary school affairs. Gabriela Pischedda[60] comments:

The term "school community" dates from the educational reforms of the government of Eduardo Frei [1964–1970]. The "national unified school" involved the parents and the community with the idea that the school would open itself to the community. Parents and teachers participated much more in the schools from 1964 until the military coup in 1973. This model was lost under the dictatorship, and the director began to be the absolute king.

One Ministry of Education official alluded to the legacy of the dictatorship in Chilean schools:

Many school directors do not view parent participation favorably; many are politically conservative because they were appointed during the dictatorship.... The law [on school governance] is very general, and there is little interest in the topic in Congress. [Often] there is no parent-school council because there is no directive mandating their existence. Many directors say that in low-income neighborhoods, families are fragmented, and the parents' workday is extremely long.[61]

The perceptions of these professionals were borne out by the author's experience in a training workshop for the JOCAS in June 1999. Committees from eight secondary schools comprised of teachers, administrators, parents, and students were invited to attend. However, there had been no systematic recruitment of parents (mothers in this case) for this training. All six women at the training were parents at the school where the training took place; none came from the other seven schools. One mother related that she was invited to the training when she happened to visit the school to deliver a note and was begged to stay by the principal. She commented on the nature of parent participation in the schools: "They call us when they want support, but we do not participate in any decisions related to the school." Other key actors[62] echoed these mothers' complaints that parents are "used" by schools. Magdalena Kleincsek of EDUK commented: "Parents are called when the grades are given out, when fees are due, or for financial or logistical support. The school does not invite them to be part of the process [of education]."

Reflection on the Evaluation Results

According to the MINEDUC evaluations, the JOCAS had the most impact within the school environment on breaking the silence surrounding sexuality, on information seeking among students, and on the quantity and quality of conversations on sexuality and relationships among students and between students and teachers. However, the data from this study and the participant-observer process evaluations noted other weaknesses in the JOCAS program besides the failure to involve parents. Although the JOCAS were a highly cost-effective intervention with proven benefits, they were events rather than a permanent resource in the schools; by nature, they need complementary interventions. Some of these limitations of the JOCAS also arise from the nature of participatory, social interventions, the modality used by the JOCAS to counter conservative resistance to sex education. The next section will show how both local and national political pressures exacerbated these limitations.

CONTROVERSIES AND CHANGES IN THE MODEL

The JOCAS Design and "Double Discourse" Systems

It is useful to analyze the controversies surrounding the JOCAS and the government's reaction to them in light of the concept of a "double discourse" system (see Chapter 1). At the heart of the double discourse system lies the chasm between a public discourse that upholds traditional religious precepts that limit individual choices and an unofficial private discourse—in conversations, interior monologues, and the confessional—that rationalizes transgressions and broader choices. Broader choices are never guaranteed, depending most often on chance and privilege.

Applying this concept to sexuality education, the dominant public discourse is the moral stance of the Catholic Church promoting abstinence until marriage even when many or most young people flout the norm. The reliance on private or semiprivate group conversations in the JOCAS program fit into a double discourse system because the content of the program (that is, the content of the conversations) never entered the public realm. The JOCAS conversations broke taboos, but they operated semiprivately within the confines of each school or community. They were neither in the public eye nor involved official pronouncements. Controversy erupted when the content of these semiprivate group conversations were represented in student murals and photographed by journalists, thus entering the news media and the public realm.

In a double discourse system, the expanded private choices available depend on mechanisms that are not universal; access to these mechanisms often depends on chance or one's socioeconomic status. This principle operated in the decentralized and voluntary design of the JOCAS program, since students' access to the program was not guaranteed. While the program's coverage of 600 schools—50 percent of the secondary schools in the country—in a four-year period is indeed impressive,[63] the glass is also half-empty. Half of the 1,200 high schools in Chile did not participate for a variety of reasons,[64] and the adolescents in many or most of these schools were deprived of their right to full and unbiased information on reproduction and sexuality. Other schools—often religious—accepted the invitation and held a JOCAS but censored the information provided. Probably more than half of Chilean secondary school students during this period did not receive the intended benefits of the JOCAS program.

In keeping with the double discourse system, the *lack of official published content* was a precondition for the broad implementation of the JOCAS, yet also another aspect of the JOCAS strategy that did not guarantee young people's access to information. The absence of any official manual or text-book with complete, factual responses to young people's questions saved the program from political battles with conservatives over the content. In response to this strategy, the conservative opponents had to rely on obser-vations of JOCAS in order to find a basis for their attacks.

According to many informants, the quality and comprehensiveness of the information provided to students was undermined by this approach. In the second workshop when outside advisors answer students' questions, their responses depend both on the advisors' knowledge and attitudes and on the degree of censorship exercised over the conversations.

Some JOCAS designers believed that it was practically impossible to censor a conversation-based model. However, the design of the second workshop in which resource people answer students' questions did allow censorship to occur. Evaluators cited instances in which community resource people agreed in advance with the school director not to answer certain types of questions or to answer them with only one possible option for action, thereby "playing tricks on the model."[65]

Most interviewees who were closely involved with the JOCAS agreed that in most instances health professionals provided factual responses to factual questions. As a result, the health sector came under attack for not adding a specific moral, religious dimension to its answers. Conservative media fanned the flames of controversy by citing numerous instances of this type of direct response.

Another way in which the effectiveness of the JOCAS could be under-mined was by limiting the diversity of resource people. *The presence of different views within the group of participants is essential for the model to function as designed.* The designers of the JOCAS assumed that multiple points of view would emerge during the conversations, allowing the process of discernment to occur as participants are confronted with and asked to consider a range of viewpoints and options.

Unfortunately, in response to the attacks the new Ministry of Education manuals watered down this commitment to pluralism. The following quote from the current JOCAS training manual (1999) refers to pluralism as an *option*, as a stance that a school *might* decide to adopt:

Since the JOCAS are organized by each school, the organizing committee takes responsibility for stating the school's framework for dealing with these topics, and therefore they decide whom to invite from the community. Besides technical competence, for some educational communities the ethical-religious position of its collaborators could be important. For example, if the establishment defines itself as Catholic, the committee could invite Church clergy or leaders (*agentes pastorales*) and Catholic professionals. *If the school community gives importance to pluralism* [author's emphasis], they could invite representatives from other churches and lay resource people to enrich the dialogue.[66]

Luckily, diversity of opinion on sexual and reproductive health matters is present in most sectors in Chilean society, and censorship seems to have been the exception rather than the rule. Indeed, precisely because in most cases the officially sanctioned, religiously based discourse did not dominate the experience, the JOCAS were fiercely attacked.

The 1996 Controversies

Following the original 1995/96 model of the JOCAS, in the third workshop (*discernimiento*) after the group discussion in the "day of expression," each student group left a written and artistic record of its reactions to the JOCAS on giant paper murals or collages, and composed songs or skits that were shared with the whole school community. This was the point of vulnerability upon which the enemies of the JOCAS could pounce, because speech or expression tolerated in private could not be tolerated in public. The murals in the JOCAS's third workshop—the only *public* moment that created a permanent record that could be photographed—inevitably generated unfavorable media attention.

In September 1996 a journalist from the conservative newspaper *El Mercurio* published a lengthy Sunday feature article on the State's "New Sex Education," including a front-page picture of seventh-grade schoolboys holding condoms they supposedly received from a health educator[67] and pictures of the student murals with condoms and contraceptive methods. One note referred to some "un-publishable" drawings, such as one "in bad taste" showing a boy masturbating "with the semen spraying in all directions." The journalist also described a skit in which a boy and girl entered a tent and "made movements and noises simulating a sexual relationship." A month of extensive press coverage and controversies followed.

In 1996 and through periodic controversies during the following four years, the three ministers involved in the JOCAS and the Christian Democratic President Eduardo Frei publicly defended the program. The Minister of SERNAM, Josefina Bilbao, played an especially prominent and steadfast role in defense of the JOCAS. In 1996, the right-wing parties introduced a bill into the Congress to stop MINEDUC from holding the JOCAS. Thanks to very firm support from all parties in the *Concertación*, as well as from the president, Bilbao, and Education Minister Sergio Molina, the bill was voted down. However, the program was successfully tarred as controversial or tasteless.

In addition, Catholic Church leaders made two requests, using both articles in the press and direct contacts with ministers: to eliminate the murals and to replace the artistic expression in the third workshop with a parent-student dialogue. The ministers agreed. Equally worrisome was the pressure to reduce the participation of the health sector. After 1996, MINEDUC assumed sole control of the JOCAS and excluded other ministries from decisions about them, while reducing its participation in the Multisectoral Committee. This acquiescence to church pressures indicates that the political costs of the JOCAS had risen to levels that were unacceptable to the lead ministers.

In the 1999 manual, artistic expression was restored but without the murals. It was still deemed prudent to leave no permanent record of the content of JOCAS conversations, even if produced by both parents and students. Murals would never again provide photo opportunities for unsympathetic journalists, thus making it more difficult for the content of conversations to erupt into the public realm. These changes in the third workshop fit into a double discourse system where transgressive actions or speech must take place in private.

Table 4.3 tracks the two waves of changes in the third workshop of the official JOCAS model through changes in the instructions in the 1996, 1997 and 1999 training manuals.

Naturally, opinions are divided regarding MINEDUC's decision to accede to the requests of the Catholic hierarchy. On the positive side, many believe that the decision allowed the program to go forward and expand. When María de la Luz Silva testified before the Catholic Church's "Technical Secretariat for Education" to describe the changes in the 1997 JOCAS, the members were so pleased that they issued a favorable report in writing. In fact, the Catholic hierarchy had divided opinions on the program, and many were sympathetic to it. Temporarily, at least, this report served to silence the most vehement opponents from the conservative sectors of the church allied with the right-wing parties eager to exploit the issue. It also calmed the fears of school directors alarmed by the news stories.

Some officials and trainers associated with the JOCAS also believed that the changes in the third workshop did not necessarily weaken the model. Arriagada comments that the students' artistic expressions often just repeated proforma and culturally acceptable slogans (like "no to abortion, yes to life") and did not reflect the richness and complexity of the private conversations. Silva notes that after the controversies students toned down their expressions to protect the JOCAS from attack. These comments suggest that the scandal-mongers in the media who invaded the semiprivate sphere of the JOCAS in effect converted the third workshop into a public space where the diverse and nonhegemonic content of the private conversations could not be aired.

With regard to the parent-student dialogue, many believe it was a valuable addition to the JOCAS. Even though too few parents participated, Rodrigo Vera of UNFPA and Silva found that both students and parents spoke their minds, leading to changed views and better understanding on both sides.

Table 4.3
Structural Changes in the Third Stage of the JOCAS

1995–1996	1997–1998	1999 Onward*
Discernment exercise for student-only groups.	Discernment exercise for student-only groups.	Discernment exercise for student-only groups but with educational resource people observing and available to respond to questions.
No dialogue session was in the original model.	Dialogue on the discernment exercise with students and adults—both parents and teachers.	Dialogue on the discernment exercise with students and parents. Teachers and educational resource people are observers and note takers to use what they have observed as the basis for future actions.
Development of an artistic expression by each student discernment group, including murals, skits, poems and songs. Parents and teachers do this exercise within their own groups.	No artistic expression.	These mixed groups of students, parents and teachers develop skits, poems and songs. There are no murals.
All of the groups view the artistic expressions of each group.	No artistic expression.	All of the groups view the skits, poems and songs of each group.
	Closing Ceremony: mainly to thank participants and to "express the pleasure of participating in this experience." (However, one of the quotes on this page in the manual mentions artistic expressions.)	**Closing Ceremony:** to thank participants *and hear personal testimonies from some,* as well as to "express the pleasure of living through this experience."

*The JOCAS manual on the MINEDUC Website as of December 2003 had disappeared by June 28, 2005.

On the other hand, many stakeholders held negative views of MINEDUC's decision to yield to the Catholic Church's requests. Indeed, it is particularly troubling that the government yielded to the political pressures from the media and the bishops given that the controversy was entirely generated from outside the school communities that had experienced the JOCAS: no parents or school administrators who had participated ever complained. On the contrary, parents and students from one community marched to the capital in support of the JOCAS, an unprecedented show of support for a MINEDUC program.

One public opinion poll in 1998 showed that the JOCAS were one of the most popular programs of the Frei government, and evaluations show percentages of dissatisfaction below 10 percent among both students and adults. The power of the Catholic hierarchy to counter these clear trends in public opinion is not an isolated case. As discussed in Chapter 1, in spite of polls that clearly showed an overwhelming majority of Chileans to be in favor of a divorce law, Chile only managed to legalize divorce in 2004, fourteen years after the end of the military dictatorship.

Would the scaling up of the JOCAS have been possible without acceding to the bishops' requests? This is impossible to answer in hindsight, but it is clear that the decision was consistent with a general pattern of yielding to pressures from the Catholic hierarchy. Often, the pressure was indirect. Silva says Catholic influence is expressed directly at the top, and ministers must face the dilemma of fielding requests from the bishops while aware of the clerics' power to affect their future careers.[68]

One observer, journalist and HIV/AIDS activist Tim Frasca, comments that the MINEDUC reaction fits into a pattern of timidity with regard to sexual and reproductive rights issues in the *Concertación* parties.

The excessive concern to find a common ground and achieve a consensus on the part of the government people involved in the construction of the JOCAS doomed them from the outset by failing to start from a rights-based perspective.... Why did they set it up to lose in this way, knowing that the conservatives do not want consensus or pluralism but to impose their position? Had the government side started out by saying, 'We are going to provide some elements because young people have these rights, and we can see how to try to respond to your concerns about this,' there would have been a better basis for resisting the attacks later.

Other stakeholders, including most of the members of the Multisectoral Committee, believed that the MINEDUC decisions seriously weakened the JOCAS model by depriving young people of their freedom of expression on sexuality and relationships.

Compromising the Right to Freedom of Expression

Some believed that the changes in the third workshop did not undermine the basic goal of empowerment of young people.[69] Others, however, saw freedom of expression as a basic element of empowerment, and viewed the changes in the third workshop as a violation of Chilean young people's rights, based on Article 13 of the Convention on the Rights of the Child (CRC). (see Box 4.2) However, reflecting the controversies surrounding the rights of young people, the CRC also qualifies this right, allowing exceptions to "protect public health or morals."

This is a crucial phrase in the CRC because in Chile as elsewhere, the free expression of young people—especially on topics related to sexuality—tends to be transgressive. It is irreverent, joking, explicit and therefore often "scandalous." In modern, urban societies, adolescence tends to be a stage of rebellion and questioning of adult values and assumptions. The caption under a photo of a skit in one widely quoted article on the "renovated" 1997 JOCAS refers to this limit on youthful expression: "The day of expression, in which the students did skits to show what they felt and had learned in the JOCAS, was eliminated this year. The young people's scenarios offended public decency."[70]

What is lost when young people do not enjoy freedom of expression? It is precisely this right that double discourse systems compromise for both young people and adults. When young people's expression is silenced to "protect public morals," adults close to them are deprived of information on what young people are thinking and feeling about sexuality. When the adults are not informed, they can pretend to themselves that young people are follow-ing publicly espoused norms on sexuality. This refusal to allow or listen to transgressive free expression by young people keeps adults at the community and governmental levels blissfully ignorant.

Indeed, one of the main positive effects of the JOCAS, as mentioned by teachers and parents alike, was that the JOCAS "removed our blindfolds" and forced them to recognize that their students and children had pressing needs for information and resources due to their sexual activity.[71] It could be

Box 4.2
Article 13: Convention on the Rights of the Child

1. The child shall have the right to freedom of expression; this right shall include freedom to seek, receive and impart information and ideas of all kinds, regardless of frontiers, either orally, in writing or in print, in the form of art, or through any other media of the child's choice.

2. The exercise of this right may be subject to certain restrictions, but these shall only be such as are provided by law and are necessary:

   a. For respect of the rights or reputations of others; or
   b. For the protection of national security or of public order, or of public health or morals.

argued that adults *need* exposure to the free speech of the young on sexuality to generate the political will to protect young people's sexual health.

Intergenerational Dialogue and Young People's Empowerment

Chile's experiences echoed global discourse and processes regarding sexuality education. At first, conservatives repeatedly insist that sexuality education should take place primarily in the family and that the state has little or no role to play. Many explicitly refer to fears that the "amoral" or "secular" modern state will undermine their religious values. However, in Chile as elsewhere, there is ample evidence that families do not educate their children adequately on these issues and that in fact most parents favor these programs in the school.[72] In Chile, as a result, the arguments in favor of public sector sexuality education as a key strategy to prevent adolescent pregnancy and HIV/AIDS finally prevailed. Once publicly funded programs exist, conservatives then turn their attention to the content of any officially sponsored educational materials and to the issue of adequate parental participation.

Promoters of the JOCAS explicitly incorporated parents into their design, not only because alleged undermining of parental authority is the most frequent conservative line of attack against sexuality programs, but also because across the entire political spectrum, there is agreement that parental involvement is a key component of programs to promote young people's health and development. In the JOCAS evaluation studies, students strongly endorsed the goal of improving the quality of their conversations with their parents on these topics.[73] Nevertheless, despite this widespread agreement and conservative insistence on a strong parental role, participation by parents was weak. The ensuing controversies showed that conflicting motivations were behind the professed goal of parental involvement.

On the "liberal" end of the spectrum, the current accepted wisdom is that positive relationships and communications with parents and other close adults are key to protecting the health of young people.[74] It is now widely recognized that programs that target adolescents in isolation from their social environment are less effective and that promoting "safe and supportive environments" is a key element of any adolescent program.[75] The involvement of parents makes programs more effective when adults reinforce the messages of the program by communicating with their children on these issues.

In spite of this apparent agreement, the differences in the underlying agendas of the conservative and liberal sectors generated tensions in the JOCAS. The changes in the third workshop are illustrative. One faction gave greater emphasis to the goal of empowering young people as autonomous moral agents through improving their conversational and decision-making skills; the other emphasized improving intergenerational dialogue between young people and their parents or teachers. Increasing the emphasis on this latter goal—embodied in the new parent/child dialogue in the revised third workshop—made the JOCAS more palatable to certain critics and led to the endorsement of the Catholic Church's Education Secretariat.

However, behind the conservative emphasis on strengthening "inter-generational dialogue" was an attempt to use sexuality education to instill a set of moral values and reassert parental control, not to empower the adolescents by better enabling them to learn to make their own decisions and receive uncensored information. Although the JOCAS model expressly includes the participation of a person from the community to facilitate a discussion of values, the writings of Catholic opponents make it clear that there are only certain values that they expect the adults involved to pro-mote.[76] The evaluation of the 1996 JOCAS noted that this tendency perme-ates the culture in Chile: "What is 'moral' appears as the opposite of what is 'sexual.' Moreover, when referring to 'morals' or 'values,' it is evident that they mean only 'abstinence from sexual relations.' "[77]

Defenders of the original model agree that values need to be discussed but that this discussion should include the full range of values in the current social context, including young people's freedom of conscience, their respon-sibility to protect their own health and that of their eventual partners, avoid-ance of unwanted pregnancies and sexually transmitted infections, the elimination of the sexual double standard, and opposition to violence and discrimination against women.

Ironically, the 1997 changes in the third workshop both promoted and undercut this goal of improving intergenerational dialogue. Although parental participation was low, the following account from María de la Luz Silva describes the benefits derived from the added parent-child dialogue in the third workshop:

It was very interesting that the concerns of the young people (expressed in the First Workshop) were completely different from those of their parents or the teachers. . . . I think the cultural gap between the generations is deepest in relation to sexuality. TV and other forms of globalized communication have changed the cultural context, but more for young people. Adults have learned that one should not talk about this topic and feel very uncomfortable . . . while the young people often think that the adults do not want to speak of this due to some psychological problem because they [must] know that young people are having sex. The adults, on the other hand, think that young people are disrespectful when they speak so openly, and they roundly condemn young people's sexual behavior. . . . It was really marvelous when these barriers came down and young people and adults managed to understand each other in this small group. . . . Such emotions were expressed! When the adults spoke, they revealed how they were educated, and this was a significant lesson for the young. In turn, the adults realized that all young people thought differently [about sex], not just the "bad ones."

Although the elimination of the artistic component of the JOCAS final session undoubtedly weakened this communication, the author attended a training session for school-based JOCAS in June 1999 in which the students, teachers, and parents *separately* prepared skits and composed songs to perform in front of the entire group. The two student groups dealt with unwanted pregnancies and abortion in skits produced independently of adult oversight. Trainers who were strictly following the official manual would not have organized the training to provide this option to the young people.

Once again, the double discourse system operated so that the "official" manual mandated a less empowering alternative while an informal and unofficial mechanism (in this case, tacit agreements among the trainers) provided expanded options for self-expression to the young people in the relative privacy of the JOCAS training sessions.

Further Limits on Free Expression

Two other incidents in the history of the JOCAS illustrate the limitations on free public expression that operate in a double discourse system.

A Manual for Resource People

Evaluations of the JOCAS had documented a need to give increased technical training to the community resource people. Ministry observers and evaluators had noted that some teachers and resource people were answering questions either with incorrect information or in dogmatic ways that shut off dialogue with the young people. The Multisectoral Committee, under the leadership of SERNAM, contracted consultants to document the most frequently asked questions in the JOCAS, as well as to suggest possible responses from technical resource people. The authors from Guernica Consultants decided to provide the factual responses to questions that demand such an answer but also to focus on the emotional and ideological subtexts of the questions. They circulated their first draft, "Factors in the Concerns (*Inquietudes*) of Adolescents on Human Development,"[78] to peer reviewers widely. The draft contained long discussions of the most common questions. Certainly one of the reasons that SERNAM decided not to release the manual[79] is that some of the "factual" responses were sexually explicit while the discussion of the subtexts of the questions often countered the religious norms espoused by the conservatives. (See Table 4.4 below.)

The document finally released by SERNAM included only the most common questions without the discussion prepared by the consultants. It constituted a minor improvement in the process since it gave the organizing committee and community resource people advance notice of the types of questions they would most likely confront and more time to do research and think about possible answers in advance. However, the suppression of

Table 4.4
Examples of the Questions and Answers in "Inquietudes"

What is masturbation? Is it bad? Why do people masturbate?	[Factual discussion]: Masturbation is not bad; it is a way to learn about our sexuality. Its function is exploratory ... . It prepares one to feel, think about and live adult sexuality. Masturbation is neither perverted nor depraved but rather a natural way to confront an unknown and emerging impulse. There is no danger in masturbating.

[Subtext discussion]: These images of perversion and sickness create a lot of tension for adolescents ... with regard to a practice that is not only legitimate but much more extensively practiced than is usually acknowledged. |
| What is the best method to avoid pregnancy? | [Factual discussion]: Ideally, avoiding pregnancy should be a concern shared by both members of the couple. ... A woman should seek professional help (doctor or midwife) to choose the best method.

[Subtext discussion]: Highlight why it is not convenient to make this solely women's responsibility. Remind participants that there is no one method that is good for everyone, which is why professional advice is important.

The first method to avoid pregnancy is sexual abstinence ... the second is to use contraceptive methods. (Next page in document gives a short description of each method.)

[Author's note: The response also highlights questions that reflect common myths about pregnancy prevention methods, i.e. douching, drinking a glass of water immediately afterwards, or having relations while standing.] |
| Is there any risk of getting pregnant from swallowing semen? | There is no way that swallowing semen could result in pregnancy. |

the full training document eliminated an opportunity to expose community resource people and all participants to diverse points of views on the most common questions. Several interviewees[80] confirmed that in fact this draft document was circulating unofficially throughout Chile among health professionals and was used in some of the JOCAS thanks to the subversive possibilities of electronic mail and the copy machine. Once again, private choices were enhanced while official roads were blocked.

A Student Essay Contest

The second controversial incident in 1999 involved a student essay contest run by SERNAM on experiences during the JOCAS. The SERNAM official who organized the contest, Gabriela Pischedda, guided the contest plans through the multisectoral process, only to have MINEDUC demand it be terminated after a media outlet gave unfavorable publicity to the contest. The announcements of the contest had already been sent to all Chilean secondary schools, and the forty students who had sent in essays were told that the contest was cancelled. Pischedda was removed from all responsibility for the JOCCAS after this incident.[81] The roots of the incident arose more from multisectoral dynamics than from the nature of the idea itself[82] and perhaps could have been avoided if the Ministry of Education had been fully participating in the committee. Again, it was media publicity—the eruption of sexuality education content into the public space—that had the ultimate effect of silencing the free expression of young people.

Multisectoral Dynamics and Demonizing the Health Sector

The multisectoral nature of the JOCAS program was one of its greatest strengths but also gave rise to persistent tensions. SERNAM, the convening agency, is itself multisectoral in nature, with education, economic development and health initiatives favoring women under its auspices. Since it does not have sufficient staff to implement programs, it is perennially in the delicate position of having to stimulate initiatives and generate cooperation among other ministries to implement programs.[83] Tension in the multisectoral committee that gave rise to the JOCAS were exacerbated by the Chilean government's lack of administrative norms to encourage such efforts. Because schools belong to the education sector, and hospitals and clinics to the health sector, the JOCAS broke the territorial boundaries.

The midwife's entrance into the school to carry out a school-wide activity on sexuality rather than vaccinations has been a turning point for both sectors: [the midwife] left the space in which she habitually carries out her role, and [the school] opened the doors of its territory.[84]

According to one official, some of the animosity between the two sectors arises from the higher social status of health professionals vis-à-vis educators. The Catholic Church's principal negotiator with the Ministry of Education, Archbishop Cox, referred to the authority conferred on the health professional: "They come [into the school] in their white uniforms, and it is as if they were wearing a crown; no one disagrees with what they say."[85]

The controversies that erupted in 1996 aggravated existing tensions within the Multisectoral Committee, resulting in MINEDUC assuming complete control of the JOCAS and their funding. MINEDUC even refused a small amount available from UNFPA in order to avoid any committee oversight.[86] MINEDUC felt it had no authority over health personnel while MINSAL had none over teachers or school directors. Thus, a result of the dust-up was a reinforcement of these strict sectoral boundaries. Many people accused MINEDUC of "taking the ball home."

Once MINEDUC assumed sole responsibility for the JOCAS, their representatives greatly reduced their attendance at the biweekly committee meetings[87] and were backed up in doing so by the minister.[88] Probably, this reduced involvement was also related to the committee members' anger about the changes in the 1997 JOCAS. The Multisectoral Committee, led by SERNAM, shifted its focus to the community-based JOCCAS based in municipalities.

Although it would seem that the Catholic Church Secretariat's seal of approval of the amended JOCAS in 1997 should have ended the controversy, socially conservative sectors continued to view the JOCAS with suspicion precisely because of their distrust of the health sector. The program's opponents then focused on reducing or eliminating the participation of MINSAL personnel in the program by accusing them of imparting "biological" information with no references to morals or values. Given the control of Chilean newspapers by conservative groups, this anti-MINSAL campaign easily found voice in the media (see Box 4.3).

A review of newspaper articles associated with the 1996 polemics illustrates why conservative columnists and religious leaders cast the health sector as the

Box 4.3
Quotes from the Chilean Media Regarding Health Professionals in 1996

[Public health] is not preserved by throwing out all healthy moral criteria...nor by systematic lies, such as selling "safe sex" to young people when such a thing does not exist....They sell them a false security in the condom preventing AIDS, and they distribute [condoms] to them without telling them what the research says, that there is up to a 30 percent failure rate. (Interview with Cardinal Alfonso López Trujillo by Pilar Molina, "Programas de Educación Sexual, Recetas 'Boomerang,'" *El Mercurio*, October 6, 1996.)

Why do a bunch of educators get together with the children to inform them about sex...and not inform them of the most essential fact: that at their age, sex is not good for them, it harms them?...The answer is simple: the JOCAS education is a disguise, and the teachers' members of the chorus for the real hidden protagonist: the Ministry of Health. The Ministry does not care whether or not the children are having sex so long as they use contraceptives because they believe that this is the way to decrease the incidence of AIDS, adolescent pregnancies and abortions. They are mistaken in this belief. (Gonzalo Vial Correa, "Agacharse, callarse y esperar que pase la tempestad" in *La Segunda*, cited in Agencia de Recortes Prensa–Cor, September 24, 1996.)

villain. Numerous religious and conservative opponents cited the typical scenario of a midwife from the local health clinic showing young people how to use contraception and encouraging them to use their confidential services. The articles also illustrate a common tendency among conservative religious forces to exaggerate condom failure rates. The commentators suggested that the JOCAS were a cover for MINSAL'S intentions to provide contraceptives without parental consent to students in alliance with pharmaceutical giants, who were eager to expand the contraceptive market. One book by Father Jaime Fernández of the Family Vicariate—*JOCAS: The Tip of the Iceberg*—expanded on the Malthusian conspiracy theory enunciated by one bishop at the height of the 1996 controversies and cast MINSAL as the dupe of forces seeking to reduce Chile's population:

Bishop Caro said Chile is being manipulated by powerful political forces, namely the World Health Organization, the United States and other industrialized nations: "[T]hey want to promote the sale of contraceptives[, so they] send their leftover condoms and birth control. There is a powerful economic and political campaign to diminish the family in our countries because the First World countries, which no longer have children, see that our countries, which have more children, keep growing, and they are going to lose their political hegemony."[89]

After the essay contest controversy there was intense behind-the-scenes lobbying against the participation of MINSAL personnel. The Ministers of SERNAM and Education met in late 1998 and agreed on a reduced Multisectoral Committee with the full participation of MINEDUC once again but with fewer participants from MINSAL. This negotiation resulted in the withdrawal from the committee of Dr. Raquel Child, director of CONASIDA (the National AIDS Commission), and Dr. René Castro, director of the Women's Health Program. The only representative of MINSAL left was Dr. Miguel Angel González, the Director of Adolescent Health Services.

Through this process of demonization of the health sector as lacking "values" and encouraging promiscuity among adolescents by offering them condoms, the JOCAS lost key input at the national level. Child notes that health personnel were advocating for better training of the resource people.

Why don't they want the topic of HIV/AIDS and Raquel Child on the [multisectoral] commission? Because we bring up issues they do not want to deal with. When we talk about HIV transmission, we are talking about very concrete behaviors that we all engage in, but they do not want to talk about this. It is much easier to say, "Oh, those poor 14–15-year-old adolescents who get pregnant and have children."...When we opposed changing the JOCAS model, when we pointed out that the community resource people needed training...we were punished.[90]

The government's reactions to the controversies transformed the JOCAS from a multisectoral initiative into two separate programs: one based in schools and directed by MINEDUC and community-based JOCCAS directed by SERNAM, with diminished participation from the MINSAL leaders in both. However, while the conflicts reduced cooperation on the national level, the health sector continued to participate actively in all the events at the local level, both in schools and community activities.

ISSUES IN PARTICIPATORY SEXUALITY EDUCATION MODELS

There is a rich store of lessons for sexuality educators around the world from the experiences of JOCAS in Chilean schools, JOCCAS in the community and replications of both in many other countries.[91] Some of these reflections on the JOCAS are pertinent to all sexuality education interventions based on bottom-up, participatory methodology.

Resistance to Conservative Attacks, and Potential for Control and Censorship

Conservative opposition to sexuality education tends to focus on the content of official educational materials and on ensuring control over the program by parents and principals. On both counts, the JOCAS program proved to be relatively resistant to attacks. The program has no official educational materials; the manuals describe a methodology and have no health content. In addition, both parental involvement and participation from religious or community leaders to comment on values are key aspects of the model. However, securing the participation of these groups proved to be challenging and not very successful in practice.[92]

JOCAS is a useful model for socially conservative settings precisely because conversations in small peer-led groups are hard to censor and because their impact relies on the power of informal, yet profound, conversation. Textbooks or written curricula usually run the risk of censorship in societies where issues related to sexuality are contentious. It is symptomatic of such settings that none of the Chilean ministries involved in the JOCAS/JOCCAS ever produced sexuality education materials.

The potential for censorship in the model arises precisely in the second workshop, in the moment when students engage in a dialogue with community resource people who respond to their questions. As mentioned above, the principal could aim for pluralism in choosing the resource people and encouraging the exchange of diverse views in instructions to these people. Alternatively, he or she could "play tricks on the model" and aim for homogenous viewpoints by limiting the discussion to pre-approved topics and opinions. In addition, there are known examples of some principals entirely cutting out the third workshop where participants interchange ideas and engage in creative expression "to avoid problematic situations."[93]

The mode of censorship does not always rely on principals. One education official noted that in the meetings of the resource people after observing the first workshop, some decide in advance how to respond to a question in the second workshop so that they do not publicly air their disagreements. As noted previously, this would weaken the model, because the JOCAS program theory holds that the process of discernment cannot take place without the young people being exposed to diverse views.

Catholic leaders showed striking inconsistencies in their support for the airing of diverse views in the JOCAS. Decentralization and respect for diversity allows religious schools to run JOCAS programs that fit their values. Accordingly, Archbishop Francisco Cox, a prominent protagonist in the history of the JOCAS, explained the Catholic hierarchy's support for the decentralization that characterizes the JOCAS: "Freedom [of each school to choose what kind of sex education program to deliver] is a risk because one cannot be sure that each school will carry out a good project, but it is worth taking the chance. The alternative is that each elected government mandates which values Chileans ought to have."[94]

This expression of support for freedom of choice by each school clashes with remarks by many conservative critics (including a remark by Cox in the same article) stating that only one statement of values should be presented to young people. The real conservative view is that the government should indeed impose values—theirs—by not allowing contraceptive information and services to young people. Catholic leaders only supported the freedom to espouse *their* values and certainly not the value of respect for the individual conscience of the young person that forms the foundation of the JOCAS.

Solutions to Potential for Censorship

Most of the solutions consist of complementary interventions. The Ministry of Health could subsidize free educational materials for young people in health clinics and in pharmacies. In Chile and in other countries where students have access to the Internet, web-based information can be made available as a complement to the JOCAS. A ministry could also subsidize several NGOs to distribute their sexuality education materials for free in community fairs held where school-based JOCAS have taken place.

Imposing Standards on Participatory Models

How, in a completely participatory, decentralized program model, can sexuality education program directors ensure quality and effectiveness and guarantee that beneficiaries have access to complete sexual and reproductive health information? How can they avoid having participants simply reflect the prevailing social norms and level of ignorance? Is guidance necessary to pro-mote gender equity and to question the sexual double standard that poses risks for both young men and young women?

Proponents of the JOCAS argue that concepts of gender equity and repro-ductive and sexual rights are usually represented in the group discussions and that as a result the process of discernment takes these new health-protective points of view into account. However, despite the rapid modernization of many societies, the Chilean experience shows that there is no guarantee that these concepts will be represented in the conversations. The plurality of points of view expressed depends on the choice of resource people and on the level of diversity of opinion allowed by school principals, as also on the existence of multiple viewpoints within the school community. Some of the key JOCAS trainers have experimented with different variations of the model in recent years precisely because they found that too many of the conversations—including those led by students—did not contain diverse viewpoints. Mere youth involvement in a program does not guarantee diversity or openness of mind.

Those in charge of implementing the JOCAS point to the preliminary training as the key entry point for guaranteeing fidelity to the model and introducing new ideas to those who will lead them. To ensure standard methodology, MINEDUC produced a series of training manuals and formed training teams in each region. Each training workshop included organizing committees from several schools and consisted of experiencing a JOCAS run by the ministry trainers, followed by an evaluation session.

Ximena Barria of SERNAM described how the SERNAM training teams found opportunities to promote attention to gender issues by injecting new ideas into the participatory evaluation process at the end of the training. A MINEDUC official described a similar process:

We promote gender issues in two ways: first, ensuring that women, both young and adult, participate equally in the organizing committee and in leadership of the event. Second, we use opportunities during the training of the resource people and the organizing committee. . . . The dialogue during evaluation allows us to remind people that some behavior that we have learned is based on dis-crimination against women.

One journalist's account of an incident during a training for the modified JOCAS—after the changes introduced after the 1996 controversies—sheds light on how the training sessions worked to counter social conservatism and to guarantee young people's right to information on sexual and reproductive health.

In Los Andes one group of students asked about contraceptive methods, and the educational and pastoral agents [priests] there refused to respond. The Ministry of Education trainers intervened, pointing out that the basic rule of this "game" is honesty. The agents must respond to questions with the truth. María de la Luz Silva, the general coordinator of the JOCAS [in MINEDUC] explained that . . . hiding or negating information [is not permitted] because access to information is guaranteed by the rights of the child.[95]

However, the extremely decentralized implementation of the JOCAS in each school increased the chances for distortions in the model. One evaluation noted the extremely uneven participation of students and parents in the organizing committees and the almost complete absence of community resource people.[96] All respondents noted that the quality of the interventions of the community resource people was uneven, sometimes dogmatic or even including incorrect information. Since most resource people did not attend the trainings, this mechanism for improving quality did not work for them. A frequent comment from resource people landing in the middle of a process for which they were not sufficiently prepared was, "How can we respond to these questions when even we [the supposed 'experts'] don't have the answers?"[97]

As described earlier, some of the internal controversies emerging during the JOCAS program centered precisely on the issue of training those responsible for answering young people's questions. However, it proved politically impossible for the State to suggest concrete answers to students' questions in any official training manual.

While the government could not guarantee quality of information or stop directors from "playing tricks on the model," perhaps the key benefit of the JOCAS simply came from the methodology itself—from breaking the silence around sexuality and stimulating conversations among peers and between the young people and adults. This intervention in itself created an atmosphere in which the participants—adult and young—actively asked questions and sought information, which in turn stimulated more and better conversations in the future.

However, young participants in the JOCAS at schools where certain topics were censored were deprived of their right to information that would protect their health. In a completely decentralized program, the completeness and the quality of the information provided to youth depend on the adults in control: on their choice of resource people, on whether to veto topics, on the level of free expression that they will allow.

The appropriate solutions for this challenge of ensuring the quality of information and counseling provided in sexuality education programs are similar to those cited in the previous section on censorship: finding alternative channels for information and disseminating information widely among both adults and young people. The solution that MINEDUC devised, "certifying" certain NGOs as sources of training and information and giving schools the contact information for these NGOs, would have worked if the schools had had the financial resources to hire the NGOs or to buy their manuals. Even while the program was still running in 1999, the follow-up funds were only available through a competitive process and were not sufficient for the demand.[98]

AFTER THE JOCAS: POLITICAL BARRIERS TO SUSTAINABILITY

The JOCAS model has many benefits and advantages, including ease and low cost of replication. It effectively breaks the silence surrounding sexuality, and the training tools are readily available. It is appropriate for socially conservative settings because it puts control over the program in the hands of the school or a municipality and does not impose content from national authorities. Its reliance on semiprivate conversations makes it difficult to censor. The JOCAS model encourages youth protagonism and leadership and democratizes the setting in which it is held. The experience almost universally generates enthusiasm and support from those participating, most importantly students and their parents. Complementary interventions can compensate for the weaknesses in the model outlined above, and in fact most of the "second-generation JOCAS"[99] include such interventions. For these reasons, the model has been replicated in many other countries and venues, including a worldwide Boy Scout jamboree. In Chile, JOCAS continue to be held without an official government program,[100] and the methodology has been applied to other topics such as drug abuse, violence prevention and environmental protection.

Given all of these advantages and the popularity of the program, why was the JOCAS program discontinued? The Ricardo Lagos government—elected in 2000—did not renew the program even though Lagos himself expressed his support for the JOCAS and for sexuality education during his campaign. The JOCAS manual was on the Ministry of Education web site until 2004,[101] but there was no support for training school teams for new JOCAS. These developments disillusioned many observers who had expected that a government led by the Socialist Party would be more progressive on sexual and reproductive health issues than the former governments led by the Christian Democrats.

The stakeholders interviewed in this study offered several hypotheses for the decision to halt the JOCAS and JOCCAS programs. Certainly, continuing controversies and the difficulties of multisectoral coordination wore down those involved. The conflicts within the Multisectoral Committee and the withdrawal of three of the members most committed to the program (Gabriela Pischedda of SERNAM and Drs. Child and Castro of MINSAL) weakened the program. Even though the incoming SERNAM officials in 2000 had leftover funds from UNFPA to continue the JOCCAS, they decided not to use them.[102] Both advocates and critics acknowledge that the JOCAS by themselves—as one-time (but possibly annual) events—are not sufficient to meet the sexual and reproductive health education needs of young people; technical advisors in the incoming administration in 2000 may have turned official attention to the need to design a more comprehensive, sustained program. However, those closest to decision-making levels suggest that the political costs of public controversies were an important factor in undercutting the JOCAS, through their effect on the priority-setting process within the Ministries.

The decisions of the incoming ministers of the Lagos government in 2000 were a natural extension of a process that had already begun under the previous government. The political will to support the program was highest in the 1995–1997 period when the President, Minister Bilbao of SERNAM and Minister Molina of MINEDUC[103] all strongly and publicly defended the JOCAS from external attacks and decided to continue with the program. However, as time went on, opponents eroded the program's financial support base from within. The low priority of the JOCAS was made clear to María de la Luz Silva who, as the person in charge in MINEDUC in 1998, had to scramble to secure funding for the program just as it was increasing in popularity.

There was no real explanation. It was just that these [extra] funds were cut as the natural result of adjusting budgets because no special program had received any increases. It was a completely innocuous response framed as part of general bureaucratic decision-making. So the JOCAS continued but with a much lower profile than they should have had given the demand.[104]

Without sufficient budgetary support for the increasing demand for JOCAS, the resources devoted to training fell and probably the quality of the training as well. Silva speculates that these minimally funded JOCAS in 1998 and 1999 had less impact than those in 1996 and 1997, which were the object of all of the evaluation studies.

Mariana Aylwin, the incoming Minister of Education in 2000, explains the decisions on the JOCAS program as a minor part of the complex exercise of setting priorities in a scenario in which budgets were being reduced while core costs were rising.[105] Aylwin was criticized for the elimination of the Women's Program, but she viewed this decision simply as part of a general effort to mainstream multiple, uncoordinated special programs under a common umbrella.

These comments point out the complexity of policy decision-making and lead to what may be the real issue—the effect of political controversies on priority setting. If a decision-maker has to choose between a special program that gives rise to conflicts with other ministries and media criticism and the core, noncontroversial activities of a ministry on the other, the likely choice is obvious. "Special" projects or programs with separate line items in budgets may be more vulnerable to cuts, suggesting that ultimately, the way forward for sex education programs is mainstreaming into the core curriculum.

Silva commented:

All scandals generate high political costs for the ministers involved.... To implement programs of this kind—with conflictive issues and strong, opposing social actors—there must be POLITICAL WILL, not only from the President but also from the Ministers who are putting their heads on the line.... There are always many initiatives that enjoy social consensus, like addressing poverty and unemployment. Democracies generate a lot of demands, and a conflictive demand related to young people does not always make it to the highest priority level.[106]

The political context for the Lagos government's decisions on sexuality education is certainly relevant. The *Concertación* feared that it would lose the next election in 2006 to the right-wing coalition, because Lagos barely squeaked by to win in a runoff in 1999. For electoral purposes, it is certainly safer to do nothing that would arouse further opposition from the Catholic bishops. Related decisions of the Lagos government in 2000 suggest that the issue of reducing political costs associated with controversy was central. For example, at SERNAM's initiative, the Multisectoral Commission took the words "Sex Education" out of its title and became the "Commission to End Adolescent Pregnancy."[107] The supposed successor to the JOCAS is a new program entitled "Responsible Sexuality," which never expanded beyond the pilot stage. Then the Ministry of Education commissioned a study on "education in sexuality," released in February 2004, in order to decide on the next steps, none of which are apparent on the MINEDUC web site.[108]

It seems duplicitous—and indicative of failure to implement a successor to the JOCAS—that two years after MINEDUC and SERNAM stopped supporting the JOCAS, the Chilean government continued to tout these programs as evidence that it was meeting its obligations to protect adolescents' health under international law. The Chilean government wrote the following response to the Committee for Convention on the Rights of the Child on April 3, 2002, to address the Committee's concerns about adolescents' sexual and reproductive health and about HIV/AIDS education in Chile:

Since 1995 the Government has been running an multisectoral program on prevention of adolescent pregnancies that holds discussion sessions on emotional relationships and sexuality (JOCAS) in some of the country's schools.... These sessions are a voluntary option for the school.... The Ministry encourages the holding of the ... JOCAS, which encourage debate on [HIV/AIDS] in the school community."[109]

Certainly, sex education initiatives in the Lagos government were designed to protect young people's sexual and reproductive health more completely than the JOCAS did, in ongoing programs as opposed to one-time events. Are they an improvement over the JOCAS? While a full answer lies beyond the scope of this study, there are indications that these programs also suffer from lack of political commitment, insufficient attention and resources. They have a much lower profile and lower coverage than the JOCAS, less media attention, and seem to be applied unevenly or infrequently in schools.

The first initiative began in the 1990s and consists of guidelines to mainstream sexuality education content as one of the "fundamental crosscutting objectives" in the new national curricula for primary and secondary school.[110] The modules for each major curricular area include content and participatory exercises related to sexuality education (including issues related to self-esteem, relationships and life skills). However, MINEDUC does not evaluate whether or not the "transversal" objectives related to sexuality are being implemented. Inclusion of the modules is not mandatory, and it is impossible to know whether they are being used at all. The ministry's supervision team only tracks implementation of the fundamental objectives of "traditional" areas of learning.[111] With the ministries themselves not demanding any accountability for use of the modules, and most teachers undoubtedly uncomfortable with the subject matter, it is unlikely that the modules are widely used. Mainstreaming may be the ultimate solution for universal access to comprehensive sex education, but the system has to include sufficient resources for training and accountability.

The second initiative is the Lagos government's new Multisectoral Program—Responsible Sexuality—that began to train teachers and parents in five cities in 2001. It is yet another special program and operates through contracts with local institutions. As the program is not integrated into core operations, it is as vulnerable as the JOCAS and all other special programs to budget restraints.

The Responsible Sexuality Program encountered significant delays in getting off the ground. Once again, the first announcements in 2000 incited worried and critical articles from conservative commentators in the media, and the final document describing the program was not released until nine months later in July 2001. One observer attributed the delays to "the typical conflict within the *Concertación* about sex. Although they know it is necessary to confront the issue, they are afraid of the polemics that arise."[112]

The program has not caught the imagination of the citizenry as the JOCAS did, nor has it achieved significant coverage in Chilean schools. As of the end of 2003, the program was present only in eight large municipalities around the country, involving 153 secondary schools out of approximately 1,200 nationwide, as compared to 600 for the JOCAS. Several critics say the program is even more decentralized and heterogeneous than the JOCAS since the methodology and content depend on which NGO or program is conducting the program.[113] A MINEDUC evaluation meeting in mid-2003 pointed out problems related to under-funding and lack of multisectoral coordination.[114] On one end of the spectrum, Teen Star, a well-known abstinence-only program, is one of the main beneficiaries. On the other, the Ministry of Health and the National Youth Institute run JOCAS-like programs called "youth afternoons" (*tardes jóven*).[115]

Lamentably, this diversity in program philosophies means that there are even fewer guarantees of fulfillment of young people's rights to health, participation and free expression than there were under the JOCAS. The leadership role for young people, which was guaranteed in the JOCAS methodology, now depends on the philosophy of the NGO or institution that wins the contract for a particular neighborhood or community. Under the JOCAS, the lack of guarantees for the quality of information provided to young people stemmed from the principle of local control; some school directors "played tricks on the model" to exercise censorship. Under the Responsible Sexuality Program, the communities covered by the Teen Star Program have censorship built in. Teen Star is an abstinence-only program that does not provide information on contraception for those who are sexually active.[116] While neither the JOCAS nor the Responsible Sexuality Program guarantee provision of the information and counselling that youth need, the JOCAS methodology at least assured a completely participatory process with the locus of control in the school and the community. In the Responsible Sexuality Program, the outside institutions receiving the grant retain full control.

FINAL REFLECTIONS: ACHIEVEMENTS AND FAILURES

Both optimistic and pessimistic narratives could interpret this story of the rise and demise of the JOCAS. Both are true; the glass is half-empty and half-full.

The positive interpretation is that the end of the government program has not ended the JOCAS. Its low cost, easy replicability, and enthusiastic reception have meant that many spontaneous JOCAS and JOCCAS-like variants continue to occur throughout Chile. All of these JOCAS-based models still rest on the fundamental premise of the transformative power of conversations. Civil society and the schools themselves have taken over; several organizations and consultants continue to promote "second-generation" JOCAS and JOCCAS.[117] Many of these models count on multiple interventions in a given setting to increase the chances of resonance in the community and to solve the problems of censorship and uneven information quality that beset the school-based JOCAS. Many observers also agree that schools continue to hold JOCAS without any significant support from the ministry although there are no systems in place to register how often this occurs. For those school districts that chose not to participate during 1996–1999 or whose request for training could not be met, this independent replication is unlikely.

Several of those who implemented the JOCAS program believe that the impact of the program on Chilean society and the school system is significant and irreversible. Before the JOCAS, many schools either had little or no sexuality education. Through the JOCAS hundreds of school directors and teachers shed their reluctance to engage in sexuality education; the conversations in the JOCAS made it acceptable to talk about sexuality and helped them to understand the need for it. They realized students could take leadership within the school and organize educational activities.

However, Silva comments that the state still is failing to protect the most vulnerable young people's right to health:

The topic of sexuality is now present in the schools, and currently only the worst schools or the most conservative private ones do not address sexuality education. . . . There is no going backwards even though progress is uneven, and what happens now depends more on the schools and the families . . . than on the Ministry [of Education] or SERNAM. This is positive because the schools are free to do what they want. On the other hand, in some schools this is a serious problem because it is the poorest children, those who most need state protection, who end up with no sexual and reproductive health education.

Despite the probable advances, a far more pessimistic reading of the current situation is also possible.[118] Clearly, the Chilean government could do better. The JOCAS experience demonstrates that MINEDUC is technically capable of scaling up a comprehensive sexuality education program with close to universal coverage of the 1,200 secondary schools. The public health system is one of the most effective and highest coverage systems in the hemisphere, so that health professionals to participate in the JOCAS would not be lacking.

Nevertheless, after the government's initial courageous public support for the JOCAS, political will faltered. Behind the scenes, the half-hearted support, the compromises and the bureaucratic obstacles that faced the JOCAS reflect a lack of commitment to protect the health of young people who are sexually active. Between controversies in the media and pressures from the Catholic Church, the political costs of getting serious about this issue are high when authorities insist on providing comprehensive and factual sexual and reproductive health information and education to the young as a bottom-line bargaining position with conservatives.

Local control of the JOCAS meant that socially conservative local authorities had the power to deprive young people of the education and counselling they needed. To counter this problem, the government should have provided enough funding to provide good quality training to a full organizing committee at each school for all of the schools that requested this support with reference materials for the community resource people. Finally, the nature of the JOCAS as a single event demands follow up steps and programs in each school to build on the openness and enthusiasm generated by the conversation workshops. These were not sponsored or funded.

Through lack of political will and fear of controversy, the Chilean government lost a valuable and perhaps unique opportunity to fulfill young peoples' right to education to protect their health. The widespread popularity of the JOCAS and the enthusiasm that they generated created a political opportunity to implement follow-up programs in the participating schools. Failing to seize this opportunity led to backsliding: the lack of follow-up support for schools that held JOCAS, the failure to promote sexuality education among schools that did not have JOCAS, the lack of monitoring of the Sexuality Frameworks in MINEDUC curricula, and the unevenness and low coverage of the multisectoral program that followed the JOCAS.

While many believe that coverage and availability of sexuality education has improved in Chile, there seems to be no reliable data to support this belief. In any case, the final health outcomes do not seem to have improved. The rate of increase in HIV infections has not slowed, and the adolescent fertility rate in 2000 was only slightly lower than in 1980.[119]

Like so many other excellent sexuality education programs worldwide, the JOCAS program was a victim of failure of nerve among the adult duty-bearers when faced with political controversies and competing demands. One factor in this widespread failure to protect the health of the young is their political disenfranchisement: they depend on adults to speak and vote on their behalf, and these adults too often let them down. Youth participation in programs and policy is young people's human right and could help to overcome these political barriers. It is commonly accepted wisdom in the youth development field that governments and programs should involve young people themselves in setting the priorities and design for programs to benefit them. Surely, if Chile's young people had had any say in the fate of the JOCAS, the program would have flourished, and continued to this day.

NOTES

1. This case uses the terms "young people," "youth," and "adolescents" interchangeably, because the students involved in the JOCAS are in high schools and in an age range that fits into most definitions of all three terms. Various international agencies use somewhat different definitions and age ranges for the terms. Most commonly accepted are the WHO definitions: ages ten to twenty-four for "young people" and ages ten to nineteen for "adolescents." "Youth"—a UN term—is ages fifteen to twenty-four.

2. WHO, UNICEF, UNFPA, 1995.

3. These meetings were called to review the Programme of Action adopted by consensus at the International Conference on Population and Development in Cairo in 1994.

4. Discussions at this session were especially acrimonious. Only after sustained arguments were the words "reproductive and sexual health" included in clause 24 of the document, "A World Fit for Children"; accessed on November 1, 2005: http://www.unicef.org/specialsession/docs_new/documents/A-RES-S27–2E.pdf.

5. See Fagan, 2001, for a full exposition of the conservative view toward interpretations of the CRC and CEDAW that support sexual and reproductive rights of young people and women.

6. E/C.12/2000/4 11 August 2000; accessed on January 29, 2006: http://www.unhchr.ch/tbs/doc.nsf/(Symbol)/40d009901358b0e2c1256915005090be? Opendocument.

7. *Jornadas de Conversación sobre Afectividad y Sexualidad* ("JOCAS" is pronounced "hō'-kûs").

8. Instituto Nacional de Estadística, Anuario de Estadísticas Vitales. Cited without details in SERNAM policy brief from 2000, and the 40,000 figure was quoted by several of those interviewed. The age range referred to is probably fifteen to nineteen.

9. In 1998 the rate for fifteen- to nineteen-year-olds was 70.2 for every 1,000 women of fertile age. Instituto Nacional de Estadísticas, Anuario de Estadísticas Vitales, 1998. Quoted on a regional adolescent sexual health web site set up by UNFPA and Guernica Consultores in Chile; accessed February 24, 2005: http://www.sexualidadjoven.cl/indicadores/ind_chile.htm#fec. The rest of the statistics in this paragraph and in the table are from the same source.

10. Chile finally passed and promulgated a divorce law in 2004.

11. From a personal communication from María de la Luz Silva in 2003:

Chile was quite a liberal country in the region until 1973. For example ... lay education was introduced quite early, with the political triumph of the Popular Front in the 30s, which was an alliance between the Communist Party and lay liberalism. [the front also had] a strong masonic influence, represented by the Radical Party, which was in power for many years, modernizing and democratizing the country. That is why I think that [one could say that] the conservative tendency, linked to the old dominant classes in Chile and which was subordinated during these progressive governments, was reinstalled by the military, transforming itself into the hegemonic power.

12. There has been an important generational change in the Catholic Church hierarchy since the height of influence of liberation theology in the 1960s and 1970s. The bishops and cardinals that were appointed by John Paul II are much more socially and politically conservative than the previous generation; see Chapter 1, in the section on the Catholic Church and Divorce Law in Chile, for a more complete description of the situation.

13. State party (Chile) report to the Convention on the Rights of the Child. CRC/C/3/Add.18 June 22, 1993.

14. "Article 24: 1. States Parties recognize the right of the child to the enjoyment of the highest attainable standard of health and to facilities for the treatment of illness and rehabilitation of health. States Parties shall strive to ensure that no child is deprived of his or her right of access to such health care services. 2. States Parties shall pursue full implementation of this right and, in particular, shall take appropriate measures.... (f) To develop preventive health care, guidance for parents and family planning education and services." Accessed in March 2005: http://www.unhchr.ch/html/menu3/b/k2crc.htm.

15. There is still no policy *mandating* schools to allow these young women to continue their studies.

16. Ministry of Education, Chile, 1993 and 2001.

17. Quotes in this and the following paragraph are from the field notes of the author's interview with María de la Luz Silva, June 1999. Silva was a member of the original design team of the JOCAS as Director of the Ministry of Education's Women's Program, and she was in charge of the JOCAS within the ministry.

18. Ministry of Education, 1993 and 2001, Chapter 3, Section 1.1, last paragraph.

19. I am indebted to Tim Frasca for his observations on this point in the 2003 draft.

20. According to a 2003 communication from Maria de la Luz Silva, until December of 1989 the school curriculum was national in scope and schools followed the ministry's lead. The dictatorship pushed through the constitutional change. The reasons for this change are beyond the scope of this study, but the military probably sought to ensure greater "academic freedom" for conservative or religious schools under a democratic government. As the Ministry of Education policy (MINEDUC 1993 and 2001) points out, this constitutional change brought much greater heterogeneity to the curricula in Chilean schools.

21. Gabriela Pischedda of SERNAM convened the committee, and Maria de la Luz Silva of MINEDUC took the lead in developing the school-based model of the JOCAS. Other members of this initial committee who took part in the development of the model included Dr. Rene Castro, the director of the Women's Health Program in MINSAL, Dr. Raquel Child, the director of CONASIDA, and a representative of the INJ.

22. Rodrigo Vera, then a member of the UNFPA regional technical support team, represented the main donor for the program and had developed this conversational model as an educational tool for empowerment and democratization of pedagogy with teachers under the government of Salvador Allende and during the years of the dictatorship. In 1994 and 1995, turning to the field of adolescent health, he adapted the model in pilot community-based JOCAS in two states in Mexico. He proposed this model to the Chilean committee, which reacted with enthusiasm. Since then, he has adapted the JOCAS models in several other countries.

23. The evaluations of the first pilots were process evaluations and monitoring reports examining implementation issues and the content of conversations. See Canales et al., 1997.

24. Luz María Pérez Infante and Pablo Mecklenburg Bravo, "MECE-High School Youth Component," English translation of Chapter 7 of *La Reforma Educacional Chilena*, edited by Juan Eduardo Garcia-Huidobro, Madrid: Editorial Popular, 1999, 4.

25. V. Espinoza and P. Aguirre, 1999; Kleincsek et al., 1998; and Abatte and Arriagada, 1998. Through various programs, MINEDUC covered the financial costs of the JOCAS. In 1996 and 1997 UNFPA supported training of health personnel to participate in the JOCAS, some of the materials and an evaluation.

26. Personal communication from María de la Luz Silva, November 2003.

27. According to preelectoral public opinion polls taken in late 1998; interviews with Gabriela Pischedda, the original Women's Ministry (SERNAM) representative to the JOCAS design team, and Ximena Barría of SERNAM.

28. There is no mention at all of JOCCAS on the SERNAM web site, accessed in 2003 and again in 2005 at http://www.sernam.cl/index.php.

29. JOCAS is the acronym for the school-based model and JOCCAS for the community-based model. Although there are important differences between the two, this section refers to basic elements of the model common to both. The content of this section is mainly taken from two versions of the Ministry of Education manual: Arriagada et al., 1997 and Abatte et al., 1999.

30. These paragraphs synthesize conversations with and documents written by Rodrigo Vera of UNFPA.

31. Hereafter, this article will refer to the "JOCAS," but some comments are relevant to both the school-based and community-based models. When referring specifically to one or the other, the text will make this clear.

32. Personal communication, Rodrigo Vera, 2002. The designers were influenced by the work of Anthony Giddens, which is summarized by David Gauntlett: "In post-traditional times, however, we don't really worry about the precedents set by previous generations, and options are at least as open as the law and public opinion will allow. All questions of how to behave in society then become matters that we have to consider and make decisions about. Society becomes much more *reflexive* and aware of its own precariously constructed state." Gauntlett, *Media, Gender and Identity: An Introduction*, Routledge: New York, 2002. (Extracts accessed in September 2003: www.theory.org.uk.)

33. Cox was later elevated to archbishop but then defrocked in 2003 for years of sexual abuse of underage boys. He cannot reenter Chilean territory for fear of prosecution.

34. "Como hablar de 'eso' sin hablar mucho de 'eso': Las remozadas Jocas del '97" (How to talk about "that" without talking much about "that": The rejuvenated Jocas of 1997) in Chilean newspaper *La Tercera, Reportajes* section, August 3, 1997.

35. Transcript from interview by the author with Rosario del Solar, Ministry of Education.

36. Abatte et al., *Texto Guía de Autogestión*, 1999, 120.

37. Dr. Raquel Child, interview by Alvaro Böhme of Guernica Consultores in September of 2000, *Desarrollo Humano Adolescente*; accessed in October 2005: http://www.sexualidadjoven.cl/diagnostico/diag_raquelchild.htm.

38. Transcript from interview by the author with Rosario del Solar, Ministry of Education.

39. WHO, UNFPA and UNICEF, 1995, 6. In some items, the wording has been amplified for clarity.

40. The data in the following table is drawn from the study interviews, and from the evaluation of the school-based JOCAS carried out in 1997; see Espinoza and Aguirre, 1999.

41. V. Espinoza and P. Aguirre, 1999; Kleincsek et al., 1999; and Abatte and Arriagada, 1998.

42. Kleincsek et al., 1999 was carried out by EDUK. The survey had a 58 percent response rate that overrepresented the results from Santiago, the capital. This was a retrospective post-test only design so that the results pertain to the participants' perceptions of changes resulting from the JOCAS. It collected data as well on the participants' perceptions of change in rates of adolescent pregnancy at each school, with conflicting results.

43. V. Espinoza and P. Aguirre, 1999. Also a retrospective design.

44. The evaluation was not designed in a way that it could reliably ascertain effects on the last two indicators, that is, there was no time series analysis of STI or pregnancy rates among students, and there were no comparison or control schools. Furthermore, it would be unreasonable to expect that a short, one-shot intervention would have an effect on these health outcomes.

45. Field notes from interview with María de la Luz Silva when she was the Regional Director of the Ministry of Education, V Region.

46. Abbate and Arriagada, 1998, 94.

47. Quoted in Oróstegui et al., 1996, 89. The following quote is from the same source. The student coordinators directed the efforts of the student group facilitators and sat on the organizing committee for the JOCAS.

48. Espinoza and Aguirre, 1999, 7.

49. Kleinscek et al., 1999, 27.

50. V. Espinoza and P. Aguirre, 1999.

51. The author heard several anecdotes during interviews, and Paula Arriagada of Proyecto Contacto has found many schools in Santiago replicating the JOCAS on their own.

52. Transcript from interview by the author with Rosario Solar of MINEDUC, June 1999.

53. V. Espinoza and P. Aguirre, 1999.

54. Field notes from interview by the author with Dr. Miguel Angel González, Director, Adolescent Health Program, Ministry of Health.

55. Interview notes, Maria de la Luz Silva.

56. Interviews conducted by the author, and EDUK's evaluation.

57. Kleincsek et al., 1999, 131.

58. Kleincsek et al., 1999, 132.

59. See a literature review of school-family partnerships by the North Central Regional Education Laboratory in the United States; accessed in November 2005: http://www.ncrel.org/sdrs/pidata/pi0ltrev.htm; Lucas & Lusthaus, "At the middle and high school levels, parent involvement practices decline," 1978; Hollifield (1994) presents a number of reasons why this is so. The adolescent has a developmental need for autonomy and greater responsibility. Families often live farther from the high school and are less able to spend time there. The organization of secondary schools is more complex, and teachers have contact with larger numbers of students. Few high schools make any one teacher responsible for a small group of students. Information on student progress involves contacting four or five individuals." J. H. Hollifield, *High schools gear up to create effective school and family partnership*, Baltimore, MD: Center on Families, Communities, Schools and Children's Learning, Johns Hopkins University, 1994 (ERIC Document Reproduction No. ED 380 229). B. G. Lucas and C. S. Lusthaus, "The decisional participation of parents in elementary and secondary schools," *Journal of High School*, 61, No. 5 (1978): 211–220.

60. Field notes from interview by the author with Gabriela Pischedda, June 1999. Gabriela Pischedda participated in the original JOCAS design team as a representative of SERNAM.

61. Field notes from January 2000 interview with the author. Source wished to remain anonymous.

62. Two evaluators and officials from the Ministry of Education and SERNAM.

63. Especially considering that there were only 40 JOCAS during the first year that MINEDUC ran them in 1996 following the five pilot experiences in 1995.

64. Reliable information based on program data on the reasons for refusal is not available, but Silva listed several possible reasons in a private communication of November 2003: fear of controversy or political opposition; other bureaucratic reasons; programmatic overload (the "Christmas tree" phenomenon in which schools are burdened with voluntary programs); previously established sexuality education programs.

65. Field notes from interview by the author with Alejandro Stuardo, June 1999.

66. Abatte, P., P. Arriagada and G. González, *Texto Guía de Autogestión de Jornadas de Conversación sobre Afectividad y Sexualidad*, Third and final training manual on the JOCAS, Santiago, Chile: Ministry of Education, 1999. This JOCAS Manual was on the MINEDUC web site as of March 2004, but in June 2005 it is no longer there.

67. Pilar Molina, "La Nueva Educación Sexual del Estado" in *El Mercurio*, September 8, 1996. The report was based supposedly on her attendance at several JOCAS. According to a Chilenet press extract from *La Epoca* of September 16, 1996, the two boys and their parents claimed that the journalist gave them the condom to hold. *El Mercurio* denied the charge. Several facts lend credence to the charge that the photo was artificially posed. First, the picture is of young boys in front of, not inside, the school, with no other students around. Second, they are primary school age, but the JOCAS was held in the secondary school. Finally, according to most accounts, midwives did provide information on contraceptives and brought with them samples of each type, but they were not allowed to distribute them.

68. Personal communication, Maria de la Luz Silva, December 1, 2003.

69. Field notes from interview by the author with Rodrigo Vera, 2000.

70. "Como hablar de 'eso' sin hablar mucho de 'eso': Las remozadas Jocas del '97," (How to talk about "that" without talking much about "that": the rejuvenated Jocas of 1997) in Chilean newspaper *La Tercera, Reportajes* section, August 3, 1997; in Spanish, the quote is: "El día de la expresión, donde los estudiantes hacían *sketchs* para mostrar lo que sentían y lo que habían aprendido en las JOCAS, fue eliminado este año. Las escenificaciones juveniles no eran aptas para el pudor público."

71. Espinoza and Aguirre, 1999.

72. There is no known case of a parent council vetoing the holding of a JOCAS in a school. One sex education program sponsored by the NGO CEMERA in the mid-1990s sent notes home to all parents inviting them to notify CEMERA if they did NOT want their child to participate. No notes were ever received.

73. Espinoza and Aguirre, 1999.

74. A recent draft document from WHO (2003) lists a positive relationship with parents as one of the four main protective factors for youth. Many other publications make the same point, including Greene et al., 2002, 60–62; UNICEF, 2002 and 2003; Kirby, 2002; and WHO, 1999.

75. WHO, UNFPA and UNICEF, 1995. UNICEF and WHO references, FOCUS on Young Adults.

76. See *La Tercera*, 1997; Molina, 1996; Anonymous, "Jornadas De Conversación Sobre Afectividad Y Sexualidad (Jocas): Una Evaluación A La Luz De Los Principios Cristianos"; Fagan, 2001; and Vida Humana Internacional, 1996–1997.

77. Abatte and Arriagada, 1998, 51.

78. Stuardo et al., 1998.

79. Although the content was a major issue, the document that circulated was a first draft and needed considerable editing to make it apt for its audience. SERNAM's decision not to release the manual occurred before the new government took office. The person who took the lead in drafting the document, Alejandro Stuardo, died in a tragic motorcycle accident in April 2000.

80. From the author's January 2000 visit. The author obtained her copy informally.

81. The JOCCAS were community-based versions of the JOCAS, implemented by SERNAM. She was offered another post within SERNAM but declined and submitted her resignation. From transcript of author's interview with Gabriela Pischedda.

82. Personal communication, Rodrigo Vera, 2002, and transcript of interview with Gabriela Pischedda. The problem was that the Committee had intervened in the schools without the knowledge of the Minister of Education because the MINEDUC representative had greatly reduced her attendance at the meetings. The Minister of Education was angry at being taken by surprise by the publicity.

83. Population Council and Overseas Development Council, "What Can Be Done to Foster Multisectoral Population Policies?" 1998; seminar Report accessed in November 2005: http://www.popcouncil.org/pdfs/multisectoral.pdf.

84. Abatte et al., 1999.

85. "Como hablar de 'eso' sin hablar mucho de 'eso': Las remozadas Jocas del '97," (How to talk about "that" without talking much about "that": the rejuvenated Jocas of 1997) in Chilean newspaper *La Tercera, Reportajes* section, August 3, 1997.

86. Church officials had also requested that SERNAM and MINSAL not be involved with the JOCAS. MINEDUC did not accept this.

87. Biweekly meetings were a major time commitment for busy and usually overworked professionals in charge of a national program. It is an indication of the importance of the program for those who originally formed the committee and designed the JOCAS.

88. Transcription from interview by the author with Rosario Solar, June 1999.

89. ChileNet Press Abstracts, 1996.

90. Transcription from interview by the author with Dr. Raquel Child, January 2000.

91. UNFPA has supported replications of the JOCAS/JOCCAS in Argentina, Brazil, Bolivia, Costa Rica, Dominican Republic, Mexico and Mozambique. The Ministry of Education has produced both manuals and videos in Spanish describing the school-based JOCAS, and SERNAM produced manuals for the community-based   JOCCAS.   http://biblioteca.MINEDUCuc.cl/documento/

jocas.pdf. Those interested in replicating these and similar models can consult with Rodrigo Vera of FLACSO, Chile at verarod@hotmail.com.

92. Several respondents (including Silva, Kleincsek, and Arriagada) reported that few priests responded to the invitations of the schools.

93. Field notes from interview with Magdalena Kleincsek of EDUK, 2000.

94. *La Tercera*, 1997. op. cit.

95. Ibid.

96. Abatte and Arriagada, 1998.

97. Ibid., 65.

98. Interview with Rosario del Solar, June 1999.

99. Name applied by Rodrigo Vera and others to JOCAS that are complemented by simultaneous community-based educational activities.

100. Some NGOs and government ministries in certain municipalities participating in the Responsible Sexuality program run JOCCAS-like community-based events. The "Contacto" project at the University of Chile, run by Prof. Irma Palma and Paula Arriagada, is a pilot project that uses multiple means, including "mini-JOCAS," to reach the young in low-income neighborhoods of Santiago; also see: www.contacto.uchile.cl, accessed in March 2005.

101. Formerly available on the MINEDUC web site. As of June 2005, a search for "JOCAS" on the MINEDUC web site yields no results.

102. Personal communication, Rodrigo Vera.

103. Both Bilbao and Molina are practicing Catholics with strong alliances with the progressive wing of the church. Silva has repeatedly expressed her admiration for the "bravery" of the SERNAM and Education Ministers, Josefina Bilbao and Sergio Molina, at the time of the 1996 controversies because they never backed down from their defense of the JOCAS in the face of media and legislative attacks. That such conduct is perceived as brave is a measure of the political costs entailed by defenders of sexuality education programs.

104. Personal communication from Silva, September 23, 2003. She left the Women's Program shortly thereafter because "I was not motivated to administer such a small program after so much effort...and so many achievements!...So when I was offered the post of Regional Secretary for the Fifth Region, I accepted because I thought I could contribute more to my government there." Unlike Silva, her replacement, Rosario Solar, did not have the status of advisor to the minister, further lowering the profile of the JOCAS within the ministry.

105. Notes from telephone conversation with Mariana Aylwin, October 2003. At the time of the interview, she was no longer Minister of Education.

106. Quotes from notes of 9/22/2003 telephone interview with Maria de la Luz Silva and from an e-mail the following day.

107. Although it seems contradictory that the same commission then established the "Responsible Sexuality" program. Possibly, the motive of the name change was not avoiding the word "sex" but making it clear that the committee would not address sex education programs in the schools.

108. The press release on the findings of the study was available on the MINEDUC web site, but is no longer there as of November 2005. The press release referred to a commission, headed by the ex-Director of SERNAM Josefina

Bilbao, which will study the results to "make recommendations on how to improve sexuality education in the schools."

109. "Concluding Observations of the Committee on the Rights of the Child: Chile," CRC/C/15/Add.173. April 3, 2002.

110. A description of this framework for mainstreaming sexuality education into the different school courses was on the MINEDUC web site, but as of November 2005, could no longer be found. At each level—primary, first two years of secondary and last two years of secondary—guides for teachers explain the important sexuality education objectives and content for courses in language, mathematics, biology, history and social sciences, English and the arts.

111. Personal communication from Rosario Solar, December 2, 2003, transmitting information from those in charge of the program in the Ministry.

112. "Alcaldes y expertos critican propuesta 'sexualidad responsable' del gobierno," *El Mostrador*, July 20, 2001.

113. Personal communication from Rosario Solar, December 2, 2003.

114. Report accessed on March 29, 2005: http://www.mineduc.cl/sexualidad/encuentro/index.htm. Link is no longer active.

115. A *tarde joven* in Coquimbo was described on this Web site accessed in March 2005: http://www.cijcuarta.cl/index2.html. The link is no longer active.

116. Description of the program accessed in March 2005: http://www.teenstar-international.org.

117. Rodrigo Vera (verarod@hotmail.com) and Maria de la Luz Silva (marilu@terra.cl), two of the original members of the Multisectoral Committee, offer their services as consultants to schools or communities wishing to develop sexuality education programs.

118. My thanks to Tim Frasca, who never hesitates to criticize failures of nerve among government officials, for the exchange that stimulated this train of thought.

119. 1980—64.9, 1990—66.1 and 2000—64.1. Data from personal communication from Margarita Pérez of the Instituto Nacional de Estadísticas, Chile.

5

CROSSCUTTING ISSUES

Although the studies in this book arose from distinct circumstances and research questions in a limited set of Latin American countries, their shared focus on sexual and reproductive health gives rise to many common threads of meaning and reflection. The clash of cultural ideas and deeply held beliefs is nowhere more apparent than in the social and political dynamics surrounding sexual and reproductive health. While the book is divided conceptually into studies of advocacy and programs, these dynamics are apparent in both cases.

These studies aim to illuminate complex social and political experiences in order to suggest ways forward for advocates and those involved in programs. In all these experiences, organizations and individuals in advocacy NGOs and in community-level programs took stances to defend people's right to information, education, and services, in opposition to socially conservative forces at many levels. One study examines the nature of social movements to defend these rights, while two others examine the local effects of participatory programs that promote a framework of citizenship and rights in the delivery of health education and services.

This chapter discusses the crosscutting issues in these studies; these include the political dynamics surrounding the most contested sexual and reproductive health issues, numerous issues related to democracy, citizenship and participation, the dynamics of organizational change, and the limitations of project approaches in social change initiatives.

CONTESTED SEXUAL AND REPRODUCTIVE HEALTH ISSUES

These studies examine experiences in putting the ICPD principles into action, a task greatly complicated by deeply polarized political struggles around three contested issues in particular: (1) access to safe abortion; (2) access to sexual and reproductive health education and services for young people; and (3) nondiscrimination based on sexual orientation. The first two issues were a major focus of acrimonious debate at ICPD in 1994. The opposition has increased in strength and intensity since then in the two post-ICPD meetings in 1999 and 2004, threatening to stymie all efforts to reach consensus each time. In these UN-convened summits, unwillingness to posit freedom of sexual orientation as a human right blocks any mention of "sexual rights" or condemnation of discrimination based on sexual orientation, and gives rise to intense debates about language on "the family" or "families."

Three of the studies in this book focus on the first two of these contested issues. Chapter 1 analyzes the "double discourse" on sexual and reproductive rights and Chapter 2 focuses on the experiences of NGO advocacy networks. Both these advocacy studies examine the barriers in Latin America to advocacy for women's right to safe termination of unwanted pregnancy—the one major cause of maternal mortality that finds no remedy in any international treaty or agreement. Chapter 4 on the JOCAS in Chile notes multiple political and cultural barriers to programs that fulfill the right of adolescents to sexual and reproductive health education and services—a right that is fully supported by international human rights treaties and by ICPD.[1]

The issue of abortion is increasingly contentious, and yet, in every country around the globe whether abortion is legal or not, women who are determined to exercise their "basic right to decide freely and responsibly the number and spacing of their children"[2] seek abortions. Even though the policy of making abortion illegal has proven to be ineffective in lowering abortion rates, religious leaders and many policymakers equate legalizing abortion with moral approval, and dismiss the possibility out of hand. Where abortion is illegal, low-income women and adolescents often seek the procedure at the risk of their lives and health, and unsafe abortions are a significant cause of maternal mortality. Those who take a public stand in favor of these women's interests may pay a price: elected officials can lose their posts, NGOs can lose contracts, grants, and potential allies, and individual leaders can be stigmatized.

Chapter 1 on the "double discourse" system analyzes the religious and political dynamics in Colombia and Chile surrounding advocacy on abortion and divorce, including the political costs for legislators. Chapter 2 on NGO advocacy networks looks at how advocacy on contested issues—or any advocacy that confronts governmental abuses—incurs costs that need to be taken into account. Facing these costs can exacerbate internal tensions, shrink the membership base, incur financial risks, and entangle the decision-making of reproductive rights NGO networks. In Chapter 4, politicians who defended the JOCAS sex education program took a calculated risk of bringing the condemnation of the Catholic hierarchy on their heads.

In consideration of these political risks, short-term advocacy strategies tend to take the route of private negotiations outside of the public eye. Indeed, Mala Htun's analysis of the process of policy changes in abortion, divorce, and family law in Argentina, Brazil, and Chile concludes that technical committees on legal reform during periods of dictatorships were often able to introduce progressive changes in laws on gender (including laws on divorce and abortion), precisely because the debates took place solely among technical experts. One of the main propositions in her conclusion is that "transitions to democracy may not lead to liberalization of laws on gender, and may in fact lead to the opposite. . . . By enabling citizen groups to mobilize and express their views, democracy opens the door to both liberal and illiberal influences on gender policy."[3]

The theme of keeping advocacy and programs out of the public eye also arises in Chapter 4 on the JOCAS in Chile. The study describes how media exposure created a public scandal focused on this sex education program in which adolescents received comprehensive and accurate information on sexual and reproductive health, and enjoyed the right of free expression on these topics. Because of the unfavorable publicity, the political will to sustain the program faltered.

The long-term goal for Latin American democracies with expanded opportunities for citizen participation is that advocacy and programs break with this behind-the-scenes logic of the "double discourse" system, so that publicly stated positions in favor of sexual and reproductive rights are legitimized among a broad range of audiences.

DEMOCRATIZATION AND CITIZEN PARTICIPATION: ISSUES WITH REPRESENTATION

Democratizing trends influenced the global policy-setting arena in the United Nations system in the 1990s, leading to the important policy advances of the consensus agreements from ICPD and Beijing (FWCW). International human rights treaties and UN policy documents highlighted the importance of civil society organization input into global and national policymaking. UN donor agencies and other influential agencies such as the World Bank began to support civil society organizations (CSOs) as part of their support to national programs, and to urge governments to create mechanisms for civil society input into development planning.

Parallel democratizing trends in Latin American countries in the 1980s accelerated in the 1990s, including decentralization of state authority.

Channels for citizen participation—especially for organizations outside of the national capital—are usually limited when all decisions are made centrally. Three of these studies (Chapters 2, 3, and 4) illustrate how decentralization increased the political opportunities for input from social movements and community members into government programs and policies, and thus facilitated sexual and reproductive health advocacy and programs.[4] Decentralization presented opportunities for parents of students, community-based organizations, and NGOs to dialogue with local authorities regarding programs in public schools and health services.

For NGO advocacy networks and women's community organizations in Colombia, Peru, and Chile, new official mechanisms for citizen participation created in the 1990s presented opportunities for influencing public policy related to sexual and reproductive health and women's health. Although these opportunities are a positive trend, the study of NGO advocacy networks in Chapter 2 illustrates problems in the ways that those who sit at the table are chosen, resulting in the underrepresentation of significant social sectors, such as rural women or indigenous women. In the same vein, Chapter 3 describes the barriers to the participation of low-income women in these participation mechanisms in Peru.

The goal of democratic participation can only be realized when the less powerful actors in a system gain more power. Reaching this goal involves simultaneously promoting changes in people's attitudes and devising organizational, political, and economic structures that stimulate power-sharing and mutual respect. The studies of the Chilean and Peruvian programs illustrate vividly how structures and programs encouraging participation could facilitate the transformation of traditional hierarchical structures in schools and medical services. The experiences in the Consorcio Mujer project point to the catalytic ability of a rights and citizenship framework to stimulate collaborative partnerships between health care providers and the people they serve. However, changes such as those shown in these programs are hard to sustain if the whole system is not changing in the same direction. These experiences from both the Peruvian and Chilean programs illustrate how "projectization" of funding leads to many promising experiences with valuable lessons, but no sustained impact.

While Chapter 1 (the "double discourse" study) does not specifically examine citizen participation mechanisms, it reveals how one sector of civil society—organized religion—has exercised a disproportionate influence on government policymakers. Chapters 2–4 describe the advantages and limitations of three citizen participation mechanisms: (1) multisectoral committees focusing on specific social issues; (2) state and national development planning committees (also multisectoral); and (3) education and health sector reform programs that encouraged community participation and/or oversight. The following sections discuss these issues in more detail.

Pressures of Organized Religion

Chapters 1 ("double discourse") and 4 (JOCAS in Chile) directly examine the political influence and activism of the Catholic Church hierarchy, which affected the legal status of abortion and divorce, in the first case, and access to comprehensive information and free expression in sex education programs, in the second.

Claiming to represent the grassroots base of the Catholic Church, the hierarchy in Colombia and Chile engaged in direct dialogue with and pressure on the highest levels of government, including ministers and legislators, to defend legal structures that deny the sexual and reproductive rights of inhabitants of these countries. Opinion polls in both Colombia and Chile clearly demonstrated that the hierarchy's stance against modifications of divorce and/or abortion law does not represent the views of the majority of Catholics in these countries. Opinion polls in Chile consistently showed around 70 percent support for a divorce law, yet for fourteen years legislators were reluctant to act on various versions of a pending bill due to the pressure from the church hierarchy. The JOCAS sex education program was the second most popular program of the Frei government in Chile, yet controversies ignited by conservative media and direct pressures from church leaders on ministers decreased the program's political support, eventually leading to its demise.

In effect, the church's pressure constitutes a violation of the principle of separation of church and state, and subverts the process of democratic representation. Not only do the church leaders not represent the views of those they claim to represent, but their pressure also causes legislators to act in ways opposed to the wishes of the majority of their constituents.

Multisectoral Committees

These committees typically include civil society and governmental participants from various sectors, and convene various governmental agencies and CSOs interested in a particular social issue. The Consorcio Mujer study identified such committees in several departments in Peru on reproductive health, on women's health, and on violence against women. The study hypothesizes that the existence of these committees should have facilitated dialogue between women's organizations and the health sector, and served as a mechanism for continuing this dialogue once project funding ended. The findings of the study qualify this hypothesis, mainly because the CSOs involved in these committees tended to be women's NGOs—which are mainly professional organizations—and not community-based women's associations that better represent the low-income users of the health services. The study reveals some of the barriers to the participation of these grassroots leaders.

The Consorcio Mujer study also reveals another limitation of multisectoral committees, which are set up in order to facilitate cooperation to achieve shared goals. When the government is violating human rights, the civil society representatives on these committees are in an uncomfortable position that makes denunciation difficult. During the Fujimori government, the "tri-partite" committee in Peru established to monitor the government's implementation of the ICPD Programme of Action could not make any official declaration that opposed the government's coercive sterilization campaigns, even though the campaigns clearly violated both the spirit and the letter of the ICPD Programme of Action. Only NGOs or coalitions with no governmental representation could make such denunciations.

In Chile, the multisectoral committee overseeing the JOCAS at the national level consisted entirely of governmental representatives; it was multisectoral only in the sense that different ministries were involved. Therefore, the committee had no citizen participation. It seems likely that the dynamics within the committee would have been much more favorable to the continuation of the JOCAS if CSOs had been part of the committee, but we will never know.

However, returning to the issue of representation, in this hypothetical case, which CSOs would have been chosen to be part of such a committee? Who would choose, and through what process? Representation issues become more problematic as the level of authority of a policy or program committee increases. These questions lead to the issue highlighted in the next section: the lack of true representation in Colombian civil society participation mechanisms.

Representation Issues in State and National Development Planning Committees

In Colombia, municipal, state, and national planning committees with seats reserved for women's organizations also provided opportunities for social movement input. The new political constitution of 1991, complemented by law 152 in 1994, established new mechanisms for citizen participation. These "territorial planning councils" had seats reserved for other types of CSOs as well, including indigenous organizations and labor unions.

However, according to the respondents in the NGO network study, these councils—especially at the national level—gave rise to problems with representation. When civil society participation mechanisms seek to include excluded groups such as indigenous people or women's organizations, how are the representatives chosen? Which leaders represent the whole movement or class of people? The traditional participation mechanisms such as political parties and trade unions that were vehicles for citizen participation throughout most of the twentieth century in Latin America have established procedures for selecting their leaders, but social movements are often fragmented and many organizations that form part of the movement have no such procedures.

The characteristics of most NGOs make them imperfect vehicles for civil society representation. Since most NGOs rely on funding for projects from foreign donors or local governments, they create a corpus of professional staff to carry out the projects. The NGOs are committed and technically competent nonprofits, not mass-based membership organizations. The staff are not elected by membership, so they do not represent any group. Although most of the NGO network leaders interviewed were aware of this issue, they still accepted invitations to sit on national or provincial planning committees representing the point of view of the women's movement.

It is important to be clear about what NGOs can legitimately contribute to such exercises. Within the framework of projects, the NGOs may have studied a problem, conducted advocacy on certain issues, or worked closely with certain marginalized sectors of the population, and so they can contribute invaluable expertise. Sometimes, an NGO or an NGO network organizes citizen consultation exercises in preparation for national or global consultations, such as the pre- and post-Beijing (FWCW) networks. In these cases, they provide an invaluable service when they analyze and report the main trends in these consultations.

However, NGOs and their networks usually do not represent the mass base of the women's rights movement, which is broader, more diffuse, and more diverse than the NGOs.[5] However, in Colombia, the NGOs and their networks were invited by the planning councils to fill the women's movement "seat," and they accepted. In many citizen participation mechanisms in Latin America, NGOs are invited because they are the most visible face of the women's movement or reproductive rights movement, and they are more likely to be sophisticated enough technically to hold their own in policy-setting venues.

The NGO network study revealed an additional representation issue: the relative exclusion of CSOs from outside the national capital. If national citizen participation opportunities do not have a budget for travel of far-flung CSOs, their diverse opinions and experiences will not be represented.

Global and Regional CSO Participation Opportunities

The NGO networks study revealed other representation problems in venues such as International AIDS Conferences and regional or global women's conferences. First, often the donors to a conference weigh in on who gets to attend, so that CSOs with few contacts among donors rarely attend. Second, global networks are set up at global meetings, so that the leadership—including the regional or country representatives—consists of those who had the funds and the time to attend. Third, global NGO meetings are usually in English, so that non-English-speakers are under-represented. In summary, the representation issues for regional and global conferences and networks are of great concern.

School and Health Sector Reform

In concert with decentralization of authority to municipalities, an important feature of school reform in Chile and health reform in Peru has been the promotion of more egalitarian, horizontal relationships between teachers and students, and between health professionals and users. The obstacles to such changes in the medical and school cultures are manifold and deep-rooted.

Peru's decentralization in health sector reform was incomplete at the time of the Consorcio Mujer study; the results of the program suggested that having authority in the hands of local officials facilitates citizen participation and enables their input to be taken seriously, producing a favorable impact on the quality of care in health services. The decentralization of the Chilean school system meant that each school director made the decision on whether or not to hold a JOCAS. Although putting the power of decision at the community level has important advantages in gaining community support and reducing controversy, this decentralization also entails uneven levels of implementation, especially where key education or school officials are socially conservative.

In Chile, a country recently emerging from a seventeen-year dictatorship in 1990, the trend to democratization with mechanisms for citizen input lagged behind Colombia and Peru. The JOCAS, however, dovetailed with a national school reform movement—"*MECE Media*"—designed to implement more participatory teaching methods, provide more opportunities for student participation, expand student-led extracurricular activities, and open the schools to the community. Although the JOCAS study did not focus on the participatory mechanisms in Chilean schools such as student or parent councils, it did highlight the effects of this highly participatory program on adult-student relationships, and the enthusiasm incited in both teachers and students by these new pedagogical models. The JOCAS put leadership of activities into students' hands, thus amazing many teachers and administrators, who saw even the worst "troublemakers" participating responsibly. The participatory methodology and face-to-face dialogue in the JOCAS encouraged new kinds of dialogue between teachers and students.

The Consorcio Mujer program in Peru aimed to transform patients in health services into citizens with rights, upending the traditional paternalistic model of provision of medical care. The program took advantage of experiments in citizen oversight of public health services—health centers called "CLAS"—that figured prominently in Fujimori's health sector reform. The passage of the new Health Law also enabled the Consorcio Mujer's work on improving attention to quality and to users' rights to find a receptive audience among health professionals. Since the study captures a transitional moment in the Peruvian health sector, it documents different responses to the Consorcio Mujer program depending on which regions had not yet been decentralized. Clearly, the sites in Lima, which the central Ministry of Health still controlled, offered much greater resistance to experiments with citizen oversight.

The Consorcio Mujer and JOCAS studies both revealed patterns of paternalistic or hierarchical relationships between government institutions and community members that posed an obstacle to reaching the program's goals. In both cases, the pattern of "community participation" was that the public institutions were merely using community volunteers when they needed them to contribute money or labor to serve the goals set by the state institutions. The community members had no input into these plans or decisions. One official in Chile remarked on this relationship as the main reason why there was so little parent participation in the JOCAS: "They only call the parents when they want parents to help finance an activity or to work on tasks designed by the school." In Peru, many community health promoters were bitter about how peremptorily the health clinic workers ordered them to do unpaid volunteer work to increase the coverage of health campaigns.

In true rights-based participation, the state agencies and community members would decide on priorities together. Adult community members would have a say, directly or through elected representatives, in the design of policies and programs that affect their lives. Children and adolescent community members would have "the right to express those views freely in all matters affecting the child, the views of the child being given due weight in accordance with the age and maturity of the child."[6]

Consorcio Mujer's strategy succeeded, at least in the short-term and in five of the six sites, in stimulating community participation and respect for users' rights. The separate training courses for health professionals and users were intensively participatory, drawing on the personal experiences of each group and demanding intense reflection on this experience. Such methodologies are necessary in attempts to change organizational cultures. The following discussion of this crosscutting theme draws on the findings of three of the studies.

DYNAMICS OF CHANGE IN ORGANIZATIONAL CULTURE

There is consensus among those who study organizational change and culture[7] that both explicit and implicit (or hidden) norms and assumptions guide the way that an organization carries out its mission, affecting the behavior of the people working for the organization. Schein provides a definition of organizational culture:

A pattern of shared basic assumptions that the group learned as it solved its problems of external adaptation and internal integration, [which] has worked well enough to be considered valid and, therefore, to be taught to new members as the correct way to perceive, think, and feel in relation to these problems.[8]

Although several subcultures might coexist within an organization, generally, there is a dominant culture, or set of norms and assumptions, shared by the whole organization. Top management in any organization can change the explicit written norms that govern behavior. However, changing the implicit norms is a more challenging task because most people in the organization are not conscious of them and do not articulate them as such. They tend to be deep-rooted attitudes and rules of behavior.

The double discourse article illuminates implicit norms and assumptions in the realm of public policy—norms that permeate the national culture, and affect most organizations in Latin America. In the double discourse system, public official speech cannot break certain unspoken taboos based in religious dogma; these taboos can only be broken with impunity if the actions remain in the private realm, and are not publicly defended as "rights." The promotion of sexual and reproductive health runs up against this system when a government aims to provide education and services to adolescents, or to promote condom use to prevent AIDS. The assumption that halts the provision of sexual and reproductive health services to sexually active adolescents is that protecting their health is equivalent to official approval of taboo behavior; ergo, official advocacy for such programs also becomes taboo. These norms pervade the culture of organizations, and need to change in order to fulfill the right to sexual and reproductive health.

The Chilean and Peruvian program studies examine the experience of efforts to change the culture of high schools (Chile) and public health services (Peru). The designers of these programs devised creative solutions to chronic problems generated by the hierarchical nature of educational and health systems, and in Chile, by taboos related to reproduction and sexuality. The Chilean program aimed to break the silence around sexuality, legitimizing the topic so that more and better quality conversations on sexuality would take place among students and between teachers and students. The Peruvian program intended to transform the cultures of: (1) women's organizations so that they would actively demand their rights vis-à-vis the health services; and (2) public health services so that they would respect users' rights. The training strategies in both Peru and Chile emphasized the learners' active participation in constructing new knowledge and attitudes—through generating questions and answers in the case of the JOCAS in Chile, and through needs assessments, examination of personal experience, and dialogue in Peru. These participatory methodologies that encourage deep reflection on personal experience are appropriate for promoting internal change in organizations.

Studies of organizational change to increase commitment to gender equity in workplaces[9] show that this process is long-term, and requires firm commitment and support for multiple interventions from leaders within the institution. The studies in this book illustrate strategies that could serve as the initial steps in an organizational change process to instill more democratic, participatory cultures and power structures in schools and medical services. However, it is also clear from the Consorcio Mujer and JOCAS studies that a short-term project-based approach would not work; the projects need to be embedded in a planned, deliberate process of long-term organizational change. An article based on experiences of training programs in gender issues and gender-based violence of affiliates of the International Planned Parenthood Federation/Western Hemisphere Region (IPPF/WHR) emphasizes this point:

While each training session might last only 1–4 days, repetition was necessary over time and change was not immediate. For example, Belize reports that "while staff members made the cognitive changes and understood the concepts, it took almost three years for the shift to be internalized and to constitute normal everyday operations." [10]

SUSTAINABILITY OF IMPACT: PROJECT VERSUS PROGRAM APPROACHES

Project-based approaches are limited in time, with a beginning and an end, and often tied to a specific funding opportunity that focuses on short-term results. Program-based approaches are strategic, aiming for sustainable and long-term effects, with multi-year comprehensive plans that address the multiple factors affecting sexual and reproductive health and rights.[11] In program approaches, any project fits into a coherent process that pre- and post-dates the project, with complementary activities that enhance the effects of the project. The time frame for the political and cultural changes needed to bring ICPD principles into practice in communities, agencies, programs, and policies demands a long-term and comprehensive program approach. The pattern of project funding for most NGOs in these Latin American countries poses a significant barrier to meeting this demand.

The Consorcio Mujer project in Peru and the JOCAS in Chile suffered from project funding patterns. An informal consortium of feminist NGOs designed and raised funds for the Consorcio Mujer project, which was the main activity of the consortium. The consortium disbanded once the project ended. Although a final grant ensured that a publication disseminated the experience of the project, there is no set of groups seeking to bring these successful experiences to a wider group of community organizations and health services in Peru and elsewhere. The JOCAS in Chile suffered from being a "special program"[12] within the Ministry of Education, so that it was more vulnerable to the discontinuities that often occur when a new president brings in new ministerial teams. As a special program, it was already likely to be given lower priority than a core program; the political controversies surrounding the JOCAS further weakened support for its continuation.

The NGO advocacy networks study reveals how dependence on short-term projects for financial support weakens the members of networks, and ultimately, the network itself. Projects that provide services to low-income women are more likely to receive financial support, while in Latin America, funding for advocacy is scarce. NGOs in Colombia, Peru, and Chile all complain that government contracts tend to have such limited budgets that when an NGO accepts a government contract, it incurs additional costs in unpaid staff time and administrative/operational expenses that are not covered in the budget. Often, the result is underpaid and overworked staff.[13] With project-based funding, most NGO staff have no spare time for unfunded activities, and many are hired on short-term contracts. However, the advocacy function of many NGO networks presupposes the availability of NGO member staff to do the work. Because of the financial vulnerability of the NGO members in this study, many networks were unable to carry out the sustained and concentrated advocacy effort needed to build relationships that could influence government officials, journalists, and other key audiences.

CONCLUDING REFLECTIONS

While the chapters in this book share the above crosscutting issues, the main shared focus is sexual and reproductive health and rights. Those of us working in this field share a passion for these issues because they touch every human being, at his or her emotional core. The positive experiences in this book testify to the healing and liberating power of communicating about these deeply personal issues in exercises that promote envisioning oneself as a bearer of rights, and that enable communication across hierarchical divides. In the policy arena, the controversies surrounding sexual and reproductive health are heated precisely because these issues provoke intense emotions. Different world views on women's role in society, on sexual morality, on dogma versus individual conscience, and on the proper relationship between religions and the state, clash repeatedly in global and national policymaking spheres and media, but also within communities and families.

At the time of this writing in 2005, in many countries and globally, it seems that the policy dialogue on issues such as women's right to safe abortion and adolescents' right to sexual and reproductive health services is more deeply polarized than when ICPD took place. This book is positioned squarely on one side of the controversies, but it attempts to increase the readers' understanding of the arguments and point of view of the other side. Some polarization may be inevitable, but listening carefully to all sides leads to more solutions.

One way to tell when enjoyment of basic rights is being denied is when people persist in exercising them at great personal cost, in spite of repression, in spite of laws, in spite of taboos. Censured speech oozes through the fissures in rigid social and religious norms, and people defy those in power to exercise their conscience in moral decisions. All over the world, women take enormous personal risks when they know that they are not ready or willing to assume the grave responsibility of another child. Young people look everywhere, often in inappropriate places, for information on sex and reproduction, and find ways to express their emerging sexuality, often at the risk of sickness and death. Organizations speak up in defense of the rights of these women and these young people, even where these topics are taboo, and suffer the costs. As democratic cultures deepen and take hold, human rights advocates struggle to ensure that states eliminate repressive norms that deny essential life-and-death choices and resources to a diversifying citizenry. In the long run, in democracies, we know that we must create policies that uphold the sexual and reproductive rights of human beings in order to create a life-affirming and just society.

NOTES

1. The Committee on the Rights of the Child's General Comment #3 on HIV and the Rights of the Child and General Comment #4 on Adolescent Health and Development; see also CESCR General Comment #14 on the Right to the Highest Attainable Standard of Health.

2. The Programme of Action of the International Conference on Population and Development, Report of the International Conference on Population and Development, September 5–13, 1994, UN Doc. A/CONF.171/13, Chapter 2, Principle 8. This principle repeats language from previous international agreements.

3. Htun 2003:172–173.

4. For a discussion of the concepts of political opportunities and mobilizing structures in social movements, see Doug McAdam, John D. McCarthy, Mayer N. Zald, "Introduction: Opportunities, mobilizing structures, and framing processes" in McAdam, McCarthy, and Zald 1996, 10.

5. See the writings of Sonia Alvarez on this point, and Korzeniewicz and Smith, "Civil Society Networks" 2001.

6. Article 12.1 of the Convention on the Rights of the Child. Article 25 of the Covenant on Civil and Political Rights recognize and protect the right of every citizen to take part in the conduct of public affairs; General Comment #25 of the CCPR elaborates on this right.

7. My thanks to Geri Augusto for a stimulating class on "Organizational Culture and Organizational Learning" taught at Harvard University's John F. Kennedy School of Government in spring 1999. Two key references used in the class were Schein 1992 and Martin 1992.

8. Schein 1992, 14.

9. Rao, Stuart and Kelleher 1999.

10. Helzner 2002.

11. One useful source that discusses this distinction within the framework of adolescent participation is: Rajani, Rakesh, and UNICEF, *The Participation Rights of Adolescents: A strategic approach*, UNICEF Working Paper Series, New York: UNICEF, 2001.

12. A special program is a new initiative within the ministry that shares some of the limitations of a time-bound project, that is, it is not incorporated into the core costs of an organization.

13. During the six years the author worked in Chile, she knew of four directors of NGOs who suffered "nervous collapse" from stress, and were ordered by their doctors to take one month or longer of bed rest.

SELECTED BIBLIOGRAPHY

Abatte, P. and P. Arriagada, "Evaluación Jornadas de Conversación en Afectividad y Sexualidad: Año 1996," unpublished JOCAS evaluation report for the Ministry of Education's Women's Program, 1998.

Abatte, P., P. Arriagada, and G. González, *Texto Guía de Autogestión de Jornadas de Conversación sobre Afectividad y Sexualidad*, third and final training manual on the JOCAS, Santiago, Chile: Ministry of Education, 1999.

——. "Las Jornadas de Conversación en Afectividad y Sexualidad: Una Estrategia de Educación en Afectividad y Sexualidad" [JOCAS: A Strategy for Education in Relationships and Sexuality] unpublished article, 1999.

Alan Guttmacher Institute, *Aborto Clandestino: Una realidad latinoamericana* [Clandestine Abortion: A Latinamerican Reality]. New York: Alan Guttmacher Institute, 1994.

Alvarez, Sonia E., "(Re)Negotiating Differences and Restructuring Resistance in the Latin American Feminist Movement Field," paper presented at the Gender and Praxis in Latin America Working Group Lecture Series, University of North Carolina at Chapel Hill, NC, 1997.

——. "Latin American Feminisms 'Go Global'," in *Cultures of Politics, Politics of Cultures: Re-Visioning Latin American Social Movements*, edited by Sonia E. Alvarez, Evelina Dagnino, and Arturo Escobar, 293–324, Boulder, CO: Westview Press, 1998.

——. "Thoughts on Distinctive Logics of Transnational Feminism," unpublished paper, 1998.

——. "Advocating Feminism: The Latin American Feminist NGO 'Boom'," *International Feminist Journal of Politics* 1, No. 2 (1999): 181–209.

——. "What State Is Feminism In? (An) other American Perspective," keynote address presented at the conference on "Challenging the American Century,"

Loughborough University, U.K., July 1–4, 1999; Spanish version of article in *Estudios Latinoamericanos* 12.

Alvarez, Sonia E., Evelina Dagnino, and Arturo Escobar (eds.) *Cultures of Politics, Politics of Cultures: Re-Visioning Latin American Social Movements*, Boulder, CO: Westview Press, 1998.

Anderson, Karen and Tim Frasca, "Lecciones y Tensiones del Armado de una Red Nacional de Organizaciones con Trabajo en VIH/SIDA: Experiencia Chilena," [Lessons and Tensions in the Organization of a National Network of Organizations working on HIV/AIDS] paper presented in November at the VII International Conference on AIDS Education in Chicago, IL, 1993.

Anonymous, "Jornadas De Conversación Sobre Afectividad Y Sexualidad (JOCAS): Una Evaluación A La Luz De Los Principios Cristianos," [JOCAS: An Evaluation in the light of Christian principles] accessed on October 2004: http://personales.com/chile/algarrobo/focus/jocas.htm.

Arcila, D., "El Aborto Voluntario en Colombia: Urgencia de un Abordaje Jurídico Integral," [Voluntary abortion in Colombia: the urgent need for an integral Juridical Approach] in *Perspectivas en Salud y Derechos Sexuales y Reproductivos*, Medellín, Colombia: CERFAMI, 1999, 14–22.

Arriagada, P., P. Abatte, C. Colomer, M.L. Silva, and R. Vera, *Jornadas de Conversación sobre Afectividad y Sexualidad*, second training manual on the JOCAS, Santiago, Chile: Ministry of Education, 1997.

Barrig, Maruja, "De Cal y Arena; ONGs y Movimiento de Mujeres en Chile," [Limestone and Sand: NGOS and the Women's Movement in Chile] research report submitted to the Ford Foundation, Santiago, Chile, 1997.

——. "La Larga Marcha: Movimiento de Mujeres en Colombia," [The Long March: The Women's Movement in Colombia] research report submitted to the Ford Foundation, Santiago, Chile, 1997.

——. "Relatoría General y Reflexiones Finales," [General Report and Final Reflections] In *La Promoción y Protección de los Derechos Sexuales y Reproductivos en la Región: Relatoría Fina*, meeting report, Santiago, Chile: Ford Foundation, June 14–16, 1999.

——. "La Persistencia de la Memoria: Feminismo y Estado en el Perú de los 90," [The Persistence of Memory: Feminism and the State in Peru in the 90s] unpublished manuscript, 1999.

Belden, Russonello & Stewart, *Attitudes of Catholics on Reproductive Rights, Church-State, and Related Issues,*. Washington, DC: Catholics for Free Choice and Católicas por el Derecho a Decidir in Bolivia, Colombia y Mexico, 2003.

Blanc, Ann, "The Effect of Power in Sexual Relationships on Reproductive and Sexual Health: An Examination of the Evidence," paper prepared for the Population Council for Discussion at the Meeting on Power in Sexual Relationships, Washington, DC, March 1–2, 2001.

Brown, L. David and Jonathan A. Fox (eds.) *The Struggle for Accountability: The World Bank, NGOs, and Grassroots Movements*, Cambridge, MA: MIT Press, 1998.

Bruce, Judith, "Fundamental elements of the quality of care: A simple framework," *Studies in Family Planning* 21, no. 2 (1990): 61–91.

Byrne, David, *Complexity Theory and the Social Sciences*, London and New York: Routledge, 1998.

Canales, M., I. Palma, G. Aceituno, G. Morales, and J. Jiménez, *Jornadas de Conversación sobre Afectividad y Sexualidad: Evaluación Cualitativa*, [JOCAS Qualitative Evaluation] unpublished report submitted to the Ministry of Education, Santiago, Chile, 1997.

Carrasco, F., "Aportes de la Sociedad Civil a los Derechos Sexuales y Reproductivos en los Jóvenes de Chile," [Civil Society Contributions to the Sexual and Reproductive Rights of Young People in Chile] unpublished study commissioned by the International Women's Health Coalition, and edited by Claudia Rohrhirsch, 2001.

Center for Reproductive Rights and CLADEM—Perú, *Silencio y Complicidad: Violencia contra las Mujeres en los servicios públicos de salud de Perú*, [Silence and Complicity: Violence against Women in the public health services in Peru] Lima: CLADEM Perú, 1998.

Center for Reproductive Rights and DEMUS, *Women of the World: Laws and Policies Affecting Their Reproductive Lives. Latin America and the Caribbean*, New York: Center for Reproductive Rights, 2001.

Chile Net Press Abstracts, "Frei supports JOCAS sex-ed program. Calls policy of avoidance 'Immoral'," *La Epoca*, September 26, 1996.

CLADEM. *Nada Personal: Reporte de Derechos Humanos sobre la Aplicación de la Anticoncepción Quirúrgica en el Perú 1996–1998*, [Nothing Personal: Human Rights Report on the Implementation of Surgical Contraception in Peru 1996–1998] Lima: CLADEM, 1999.

Consorcio Mujer, *Calidad de Atención en la Salud Reproductiva: Una Mirada desde la Ciudadanía Feminina*, [Quality of care in reproductive health: From the perspective of women's citizenship] Lima, Peru: Consorcio Mujer, 1998.

——. *Compromiso para Fortalecer la Participación Ciudadana desde los Servicios de Salud: Modulo de Capacitación a Personal de los Servicios de Salud*, [The health services' commitment to strengthen citizen participation: Training manual for health service providers] Lima, Peru: Consorcio Mujer, 2000.

——. *Fortaleciendo las Habilidades Ciudadanas de las Mujeres en Salud: Modulo de Capacitación a Líderes de Salud*, [Strengthening women's citizenship skills in health: Training manual for health leaders] Lima, Peru: Consorcio Mujer, 2000.

——. *Se Hace Camino al Andar: Aportes a la Construcción de la Ciudadania de las Mujeres en Salud*, [Forging paths: Resources for the construction of women's citizenship in health] Lima, Peru: Consorcio Mujer, 2000.

Dunlop, Joan, Rachel Kyte, and Mia MacDonald, "Women Redrawing the Map: The World after the Beijing and Cairo Conferences," *SAIS Review* 16, No. 1 (Winter-Spring 1996).

Espinoza, V. and P. Aguirre, "Evaluación de Impacto de las Jornadas de Conversación sobre Afectividad y Sexualidad," [Evaluation of the Impact of the Conversation Workshops on Relationships and Sexuality] executive summary of Evaluation Report on the 1997 JOCAS, Santiago, Chile: Ministry of Education, 1999.

Fagan, Patrick F., "How U.N. Conventions on Women's and Children's Rights Undermine Family, Religion, and Sovereignty," *The Heritage Foundation Backgrounder 1407*, February 5, 2001.

FOCUS on Young Adults, *Advancing Young Adult Reproductive Health: Actions For the Next Decade*, Washington, DC: Pathfinder International, The Futures Group International, and Tulane University School of Health and Tropical Medicine, 2001.

Ford Foundation and ICMER, "La Promoción y Protección de los Derechos Sexuales y Reproductivos en la Región: Relatoría Final," [Promotion and Protection of Sexual and Reproductive Rights in the Region: Final Report] report of a meeting held in Santiago, Chile: Ford Foundation and ICMER, June 14–16, 1999.

Foweraker, Joe, "Theorizing Social Movements," In *Critical Studies on Latin America Series*, edited by Jenny Pearce, London and Boulder, CO: Pluto Press, 1995.

Freire, Paulo, *Pedagogy of the Oppressed*, New York: Continuum, 1986 [1970].

Gamson, William A., *The Strategy of Social Protest*, Belmont, CA: Wadsworth Publishers, 1990.

Gilligan, Carol, *In a Different Voice: Psychological Theory and Women's Development*, Cambridge, MA: Harvard University Press, 1993 [1982].

Girard, Françoise, "Cairo+Five: Reviewing Progress for Women Five Years after the International Conference on Population and Development," Journal *of Women's Health and Law* 1, No. 1 (November 1999): 1–14.

Greene, M., Z. Rasekh, and K. Amen, *In This Generation: Sexual and Reproductive Health Policies for a Youthful World*, Washington, DC: Population Action International, 2002.

Greig, Alan, Michael Kimmel, and James Lang, "Men, Masculinities and Development: Broadening our work towards gender equality," UNDP/GIDP, *Monograph* 10, 2000.

Grupo Impulsor Nacional, *Mujeres y Ciudadanía en el Perú: Avances y Barreras*, [Women and Citizenship in Peru: Advances and Obstacles] Lima, Peru: Grupo Impulsor Nacional, 1998.

Gruskin, Sofia (ed.) "Special Focus: Women's Health and Human Rights," *Health and Human Rights* 1, No. 4, 1995.

———. "The Conceptual and Practical Implications of Reproductive and Sexual Rights: How Far Have We Come?" *Health and Human Rights* 4, No. 2 (2000): 1–6.

Gruskin, Sofia, Michael A. Grodin, George J. Annas, and Stephen P. Marks, (eds.) *Perspectives on Health and Human Rights*, New York: Routledge, 2005.

Guedes, Allesandra, Lynne Stevens, Judith F. Helzner, and Susanna Medina, "Integrating Gender-Based Violence into A Reproductive and Sexual Health Program in Venezuela," in *Responding to Cairo: Case studies of changing practice in reproductive health and family planning*, edited by N. Haberland and D. Measham, New York: Population Council, 2002.

Guedes, Allesandra, S. Bott, Ana Guezmes, and Judith F. Helzner, "Gender-based violence, human rights and the health sector: Lessons from Latin America," *Health and Human Rights* 6, No. 1, 2002.

Guernica Consultores S.A., "Monitoring and Evaluation Plan on the Quality of the JOCCAS," (*Plan de Monitoreo y Evaluación de Calidad de las JOCCAS*) executive summary (author, Alejandro Stuardo) and first and second Interim reports; (*Resumen Ejecutivo y Primero y Segunda Informes de Avance.*) unpublished first draft of evaluation commissioned by the Intersectorial Commission on Sexual Education and Prevention of Adolescent Pregnancy. Santiago, Chile: Guernica Consultores, 1998.

Haberland, Nicole and Diana Measham (eds.) *Responding to Cairo: Case studies of changing practice in reproductive health and family planning*, New York: The Population Council, 2002.

Hass, L., "The Catholic Church in Chile,' in C. Smith and J. Prokopy (eds.) *Latin American Religion in Motion*," New York and London: Routledge, 1999.

Helzner, Judith F. and Bonnie L. Shepard, "The Feminist Agenda in Population Private Voluntary Organizations," *Women, International Development, and Politics: The Bureaucratic Mire*, edited by Kathleen Staudt, Philadelphia: Temple University Press, 1990 and 1997.

Helzner, Judith F., "Transforming family planning services in the Latin American and Caribbean region," *Studies in Family Planning* 33, No. 1 (2002): 49–60.

Hola, Eugenia and Ana María Portugal (eds.) *La Ciudadanía a Debate* [Debates on citizenship], Ediciones de las Mujeres No. 25, Santiago, Chile: ISIS Internacional and CEM, 1997.

Hord, Charlotte E., *Construir acceso al aborto seguro: Una guía práctica para el Advocacy* [Constructing access to safe abortion: A practical advocacy guide], Chapel Hill, NC: IPAS, 2002.

Htun, Mala, *Sex and the State: Abortion, Divorce, and the Family under Latin American Dictatorships and Democracies*, Cambridge, UK: Cambridge University Press, 2003.

Hula, Kevin W., *Lobbying Together: Interest Group Coalitions in Legislative Politic*, American Governance and Public Policy Series, edited by Barry Rabe and John Tierney, Washington, DC: Georgetown University Press, 1999.

International Council of AIDS Service Organizations (ICASO), *Manual para el Trabajo en Red sobre VIH/SIDA*, Toronto: ICASO, 1997.

International Planned Parenthood Federation, Western Hemisphere Region (IPPF/WHR), *Manual to Evaluate Quality of Care from a Gender Perspective*, New York, IPPF/WHR, 2000.

Jelin, Elizabeth, "Toward a Culture of Participation and Citizenship," In *Cultures of Politics, Politics of Cultures: Re-Visioning Latin American Social Movements*, edited by Sonia E. Alvarez, Evelina Dagnino and Arturo Escobar, Boulder, CO: Westview Press, 1998.

Keck, Margaret E. and Kathryn Sikkink, *Activists beyond Borders: Advocacy Networks in International Politics*, Ithaca, NY and London: Cornell University Press, 1998.

Kingslow Associates, "Factors Affecting the Growth and Effectiveness of Reproductive Rights Coalitions: An Assessment Prepared for the Ms. Foundation for Women," unpublished report, 1998.

Kirby, Douglas, *Emerging Answers: Research Findings on Programs to Reduce Sexual Risk-Taking and Teen Pregnancy*, Washington, DC: The National Campaign to Prevent Teen Pregnancy, 2001.

Kleincsek, Magdalena, G. Guajardo, D. Rivera, and V. Espinoza, "Informe Final: Evaluación del Impacto de Largo Plazo de las Jornadas de Conversación sobre Afectividad y Sexualidad (JOCAS) en la Comunidad Educativa y las Familias en las Regiones IV, VII y Metropolitana (1996)," [Final Report of the Long-term Impact Evaluation of the JOCAS] unpublished report to the Ford Foundation. Santiago, Chile: EDUK, 1999.

Korzeniewicz, Roberto P. and William C. Smith, *Protest and Collaboration: Transnational Civil Society Networks and the Politics of Summitry and Free Trade in the Americas.* North-South Agenda Paper 51 (September), Coral Gables, FL: The Dante B. Fascell North-South Center at the University of Miami, 2001.

———. "Civil Society Networks: The Old and New Politics of Representation in Latin America," paper prepared for the collaborative conferences on "Representation and Democratic Politics in Latin America" organized by the Universidad de San Andrés, Victoria, Argentina, on June 7–8, 2001, and by the University of Pittsburgh on September 4, 2001.

Kuhn, Thomas, *The Structure of Scientific Revolutions*, Chicago, IL:University of Chicago Press, 1962.

Lamas, Marta, *Política y Reproducción Aborto: La Frontera del Derecho a Decidir*, Barcelona and Mexico City: Plaza y Janés, 2001.

Lightfoot, Sarah Lawrence, *The Art and Science of Portraiture*, San Francisco: Jossey Bass Publishers, 1997.

Martin, Joanne, *Cultures in Organizations: Three Perspectives*, Oxford: Oxford University Press, 1992.

Marwell, Gerald, Pamela Oliver, and Ralph Prahl, "Social Networks and Collective Action: A Theory of the Critical Mass. III," *American Journal of Sociology* 84 (1988): 1335–1360.

McAdam, Doug, John D. McCarthy, and Mayer N. Zald (eds.) *Comparative Perspectives in Social Movements: Political Opportunities, Mobilizing Structures, and Cultural Framings*, 2nd ed., Cambridge, UK: Cambridge University Press, 1996.

Miller, Alice M., "Sexual but Not Reproductive: Exploring the Junction and Disjunction of Sexual and Reproductive Rights," *Health and Human Rights* 4, No. (2000): 68–109.

Ministerio de Salud and USAID, "Los primeros años del proyecto 2000: 1993–1997" [The First years of Project 2000: 1993–1997] Lima, Peru: Ministerio de Salud, 1997.

Ministry of Education, "Política de Educación en Sexualidad: Para el Mejoramiento de la Calidad de la Educación," [Policy on Sexuality Education: For the Improvement of the Quality of Education] Santiago, Chile: Ministry of Education, 1993 and 2001.

Mische, Ann and Philippa Pattison, "Composing a Civic Arena: Publics, Projects, and Social Settings," *Poetics* 27 (2000): 163–194.

Molina, Pilar, "La Nueva Educación Sexual del Estado," [The State's New Sex Education] *El Mercurio*, September 8, 1996.

National Statistics Institute, *National Household Survey (ENAHO) of the National Statistics Institute (INEI) 4th quarter, 1995 and 1997*, Lima, Peru: National Statistics Institute, 1999.

——- *Encuesta Demográfica y de Salud Familiar 2000*, [Demographic and family health survey 2000] Lima, Peru: National Statistics Institute, 2000.

Olson, Mancur, *The Logic of Collective Action*, Cambridge, MA: Harvard University Press, 1965.

Oré Aguilar, Gaby, "Introducción," In "La Promoción y Protección de los Derechos Sexuales y Reproductivos en la Región: Relatoría Final," report of a meeting held in Santiago, Chile: Ford Foundation and ICMER, June 14–16, 1999.

Oróstegui, Ina, M. Kleinscek, P. Abatte, G. González, and P. Arriagada, *Jornadas de Conversación sobre Afectividad y Sexualidad 96*, first training manual on the JOCAS, Santiago, Chile: Ministry of Education, Women's Program, 1996.

Patel, Mahesh, "Human Rights as an Emerging Development Paradigm and Some Implications for Programme Planning, Monitoring and Evaluation," draft paper presented at UNICEF Global Consultation on Human Rights Approach to Programming, Tanzania, August 5–8, 2002.

Pehrsson, Kajsa, Siv Näslund, and Marianne Bull, "Evaluation of Women's Networks Supported by the Nordic Countries: A Consultancy Report," Development Studies Unit, Department of Social Anthropology, Stockholm University, 1990.

Petchesky, Rosalind, "Rights and Needs: Rethinking the Connections in Debates over Reproductive and Sexual Rights," *Health and Human Rights* 4, No. 2, (2000): 17–30.

Poniatowska, Elena, *Las mil y una ... (la herida de Paulina)*, [A thousand and one ... (Paulina's wound)] Mexico City, Mexico: Plaza y Janés, 2000.

Population Council and Population Reference Bureau, "A Guide to Research Findings on the Cairo Consensus," New York: Population Council, 1999.

Presidencia de la Republica, *Plan Nacional de Población: 1998–2002*, [Nacional Population Plan] Lima, Peru: PROMUDEH, 1998.

Rajani, Rakesh and UNICEF, *The Participation Rights of Adolescents: A strategic approach*, UNICEF Working Paper Series, New York: UNICEF, 2001.

Rao, Aruna, Rieky Stuart, and David Kelleher, *Gender at Work: Organizational Change for Equality*, West Hartford, CT: Kumarian Press, 1999.

Robey, Bryant and Megan Drennan, "La participación en la salud de la reproducción," [The Participation of Health in Reproduction] *Network en Español* 18, No. 3 (Primavera [Spring] 1998): 12–17.

Rose, Fred, *Coalitions across the Class Divide: Lessons from the Labor, Peace, and Environment Movements*, Ithaca, NY: Cornell University Press, 2000.

Royal Tropical Institute, *Institutionalizing Gender Equality*, Amsterdam, the Netherlands: Royal Tropical Institute and Oxfam, GB, 2000.

Salamon, Lester, Helmut K. Anheier, Regina List, Stefan Toepler, S. Wojciech Sokolowski and Associates, *Global Civil Society: Dimensions of the Nonprofit Sector*, Baltimore, MD: Center for Civil Society Studies, 1999.

Sanborn, Cynthia, "The Fabric of Civil Society? Philanthropy and Nonprofits in Latin America," paper presented in a workshop on "Regulatory Reform, Philanthropy, and Social Change in Latin America," sponsored by the David Rockefeller Center for Latin American Studies and the Hauser Center for Nonprofit Organizations, at Harvard University on March 13–14, 2000.

Schein, Edgar H., *Organizational Culture and Leadership*, New York: Jossey-Bass, Inc, 1992.

Shepard, Bonnie L., "Addressing Gender Issues with Men and Couples: Involving Men in Sexual and Reproductive Health Services in APROFE, Ecuador," *International Journal of Men's Health* 3, No. 3 (2005): 155–172.

Shepard, Bonnie L., "The 'Double Discourse' on Sexual and Reproductive Rights: The Chasm between Public Policy and Private Actions." *Health and Human Rights* 4, No. 2 (2000): 110–143.

——. "Let's Be Citizens, Not Patients: Women's Groups in Peru Assert Their Right to High-Quality Reproductive Health Care," In *Responding to Cairo: Case Studies of Changing Practice in Reproductive Health and Family Planning*, edited by Nicole Haberland and Diana Measham, New York: The Population Council, 2002.

——. *NGO Advocacy Networks in Latin America: Lessons from Experience in Promoting Women's and Reproductive Rights in Latin America.* North-South Agenda Paper 61 of The Dante B. Fascell North-South Center at the University of Miami, Miami, FL, 2003.

——. " 'When I talk about sexuality, I use myself as an example': Sexuality counseling and family planning in Colombia," in *Responding to Cairo: Case studies of changing practice in reproductive health and family planning*, edited by Nicole Haberland and Diana Measham, New York: The Population Council, 2002.

——. "Reproductive Health: Building Women's Citizenship" in *DRCLAS News*, Fall 2000, special issue on Health and Equity in the Americas, published by the David Rockefeller Center for Latin American Studies, Harvard University; accessed on October 2005: http://drclas.fas.harvard.edu/revista/?issue_id=6.

Shepard, Bonnie, L. José García Nuñez and Saul Helfenbein, "Youth Program Strategies in the Bill and Melinda Gates Foundation's Global Health Program," unpublished report, 2000.

Silliman, Jael, "Expanding Civil Society, Shrinking Political Spaces: The Case of Women's Nongovernmental Organizations," in *Dangerous Intersections: Feminist Perspectives on Population, Environment and Development*, edited by Jael Silliman and Ynestra King, Boston, MA: South End Press, 1999.

Smith, C. and J. Prokopy (eds.) *Latin American Religion in Motion*, New York and London: Routledge, 1999.

Stake, Robert E., *The Art of Case Study Research*, Thousand Oaks, CA: Sage Publications, 1995.

Stuardo, Alejandro, Maria Pía Oliveira, and Alvaro Böhme, "Material de Apoyo para Agentes Educativos: Elementos para el Reconocimiento de Inquietudes adolescentes en Desarrollo Humano," [Support materials for educational agents: Elements to Recognize Adolescents' Concerns on Human Development] unpublished draft submitted to SERNAM and distributed to peer reviewers, 1998.

Stuardo, Alejandro, "Informe Final: Sistematización de rasgos socio políticos y culturales en que se contextualiza el primer estudio nacional de comportamiento sexual en Chile," [Final Report: Systematic analysis of the socio-political and cultural aspects of the context of the first national study of sexual behavior in Chile] draft of unfinished report to SERNAM, 2000.

Swedish International Development Cooperation Agency (SIDA), *Webs Women Weave: A Synthesis Report on Four Organisations Working with Sexual and*

Reproductive Health and Rights, Stockholm, Sweden: SIDA, Department for Democracy and Social Development, Health Division, 2000.

Ugarte, Oscar and José Antonio Monje, "Equidad y reforma en el sector salud," [Equity and reform in the health sector] unpublished paper, Lima, Peru: Universidad del Pacífico, 1999.

UNAIDS, *Report on the Global HIV/AIDS Epidemic*, Geneva: 2000.

UNAIDS, Vargas, Hernán A., José Bernardo Toro A. and Martha C. Rodríguez G., *Acerca de la Naturaleza y Evolución de los Organismos no Gobernamentales (ONGs) en Colombia*, [The Characteristics and the Evaluation of the NGOs in Colombia] Santafé de Bogotá: Fundación Social, 1992.

UNICEF, *Human rights for children and women: How UNICEF helps to make them a reality*, New York: UNICEF, 1999.

——. "Programme Working Note: HIV Prevention among Young People," draft, 2002.

——. "Programming for Adolescence," draft technical paper, June 2003.

UNICEF, UNAIDS, WHO, *Young People and HIV/AIDS: Opportunity in Crisis*, accessed on October 2005: http://www.unicef.org/publications/files/pub_youngpeople_hivaids_en.pdf. 2002.

United Nations, "Core document forming part of the reports of states parties: Peru," submitted to the UN treaty bodies, HRI/CORE/1/Add.43/Rev1.

Valdés, Teresa and José Olavarría (eds.) *Masculinidades y equidad de género en América Latina*, [Masculinities and Gender Equity in Latin America] Santiago, Chile: FLACSO-Chile, 2003.

Vargas, Hernán A., José Bernardo Toro A., *et al.*, *Acerca de la Naturaleza y Evolución de los Organismos no Gobernamentales (ONGs) en Colombia*, Santafé de Bogotá, Colombia: Fundación Social, 1992.

Vera, Rodrigo, "Jornadas de Conversación sobre Afectividad y Sexualidad: JOCAS. Experiencia del Gobierno Chileno," [JOCAS: The Experience of the Chilean Government] unpublished report, UNFPA, Equipo de Apoyo Técnico del UNFPA para América Latina y el Caribe, 1997.

Vida Humana Internacional, "Escoge La Vida," [Choose Life] *Boletín* 64 (Nov. 1996–Feb. 1997).

Watts, Jerry Gafio, "Blacks and Coalition Politics: A Theoretical Reconceptualization," in *The Politics of Minority Coalitions: Race, Ethnicity, and Shared Uncertainties*, edited by Wilbur C. Rich, Westport, CT: Praeger, 1996.

WHO, UNFPA and UNICEF, "Action for Adolescent Health: Towards a Common Agenda," WHO/FRH/ADH/97.9; accessed on October 2005: http://www.who.int/child-adolescent-health/New_Publications/ADH/WHO_FRH_ADH_97.9_en.pdf, 1995.

WHO, Adolescent Health and Development Programme, *Risk and Protective Factors affecting Adolescent Health and Development*, Geneva & New York: WHO/UNICEF. Ref. WHO/FCH/CAH/00.20, 1999.

WHO, Department of Child and Adolescent Health and Development, "Broadening the Horizon: Balancing Protection and Risk for Adolescents," draft document, June 2003.

Wisely, Nancy, "Social Movements," in *Political Networks: The Structural Perspective*, edited by David Knoke, New York: Cambridge University Press, 1990.

INDEX

About the Author

BONNIE SHEPARD is a researcher and program evaluator affiliated with the International Health and Human Rights Program at Harvard University School of Public Health.